Mourning Sarah

a case for testing group B strep

Contents

Foreword

No one realized Sarah Vigour, just hours old, was sick. Not until she was very sick with sepsis. In less than a day an undetected group B streptococcus (GBS) infection claimed the little one's life.

Theresa Vigour, her mother, has carried the memory of that day since 1981. Twenty-seven years later, she has preserved Sarah's story on these superbly written pages – every hopeful, tender, terrifying, angry, grief-filled moment of it. *Mourning Sarah* is filled with important, even urgent, messages for any woman having a baby right here, right now, and for all young girls who soon will grow into womanhood and want babies of their own.

The first message of the story is the enduring bond between a bereaved mother and her infant. While Western culture still tacitly encourages us to forget and move on, every bereaved parent of a baby knows the day of birth, or stillbirth, is the first in a lifelong love relationship. A birth is a birth, no matter the outcome. A child is a child, alive or dead. To forget a child is impossible.

But Sarah's story has another message: it raises consciousness about GBS. While Western culture soothes itself with the notion that survival of the fittest is a good thing for the human race, the reality is that many GBS babies are fit, save for the undetected bacterium. In 1999 my daughter, Victoria, stricken by this silent and symptomless killer at 42 weeks of pregnancy, was stillborn. The infection caused her to aspirate meconium, according to her autopsy. Otherwise, she was a healthy and beautiful child with perfectly formed crimson lips, a pretty face, dainty hands and feet – the love of my life.

Theresa Vigour articulates the unspeakable loss of her daughter using every hue in the emotional rainbow. Her account is exquisite, her metaphors masterful, and throughout the book, she skillfully weaves her inner and outer worlds. As grief engulfs her, for instance, she describes her surroundings as surreal, foggy and gray, contrasting with the lush, colorful world of her coastal North Carolina home.

Though *Mourning Sarah* is foremost a human drama, Theresa Vigour also offers an easy-to-follow and startling history of GBS, a history that moves and amazes readers all the more because it is set against the backdrop of her daughter's short life. That history starts in 1938, the year the link between GBS and neonatal disease was first made. As of this writing, GBS is still a leading infectious killer of newborns and the leading cause of blood infection and meningitis in newborns, according to Group B Strep International.

Since 1996 when the Centers for Disease Control (CDC) first issued guidelines to prevent GBS disease in babies, American mothers have been tested for the presence of the bacterium. The culture test – quick, inexpensive and performed around the 35th week of pregnancy – has saved many lives. Before active intervention, some 7500 American babies got GBS disease every year. Today those numbers have improved because if a mother tests positive, she is monitored and antibiotics are administered to avert tragedy.

But testing once is not enough. For the past four years I have encountered many mothers nationwide who, like me, tested negative for GBS around the 35th week. But the bacterium appeared later in the pregnancy, when there is no testing and so no detection. Similarly, administering just one test imperils premature babies who are delivered before the 35th week.

Make no mistake about it, even mothers are imperiled by the bacterium. Nine years ago GBS almost killed me. I felt fine when I entered an operating room for a C-section and emerged with a dead child and a 103° fever that fluctuated but did not quit for some 15 days. Finally, my doctor located and eradicated the last of the GBS in my body.

GBS is not going away. But thousands of American babies already have. *Mourning Sarah* has the power to help keep alive the momentum to test well and frequently, a momentum propelled in the United States by parent activists. I hope Sarah's story similarly helps a movement already begun in England to test mothers in its National Health Service where, I am told, there is no testing done at all.

GBS is not a conundrum. It is not a mystery. It is a problem that comes complete with a solution: constant testing of pregnant women. So what prevents this constant testing from taking place? Fear and ignorance. In this book Theresa Vigour talks about her old fears evaporating in the wake of her daughter's death.

She pushed through her fears about going back to school, about having another child, and many more.

Individually, we each need to summon that kind of courage to break through the barrier of personal fear and denial that stops parents from asking for, and even thinking about, GBS tests. Culturally, we need to find the will to use all the knowledge and resources we already have to help infants who, were it not for GBS, would live healthy lives. We did not do that for Sarah Vigour or for Victoria Ash or for thousands of others. These babies are not statistics. They are not case studies. They are our irreplaceable daughters and sons.

Theresa Vigour has given us a gift. She has borne witness to an important pivot point in the history of birthing. We all would do well to look where she directs our attention and then show enough character as a civilization to love and save our most vulnerable citizens – the babies of generations yet to come. To do so is to create a better and more compassionate world and to honor the memory of babies such as Sarah Vigour, already lost but no less loved.

Lorraine Ash
Author, *Life Touches Life: A Mother's Story*
of Stillbirth and Healing

Foreword

I was five years old when I met my sister, Sarah, in a picture while she and Mom were still in the hospital. Her head full of red hair was cradled in Mom's hand with the hospital wristband visible. I had looked forward to being a big sister but her death robbed me of that role. Her death probably influenced my career choice. I chose medicine, so I can heal, cure, and comfort my patients. I wanted to be in a doctor–patient relationship where I would watch children grow from the first newborn exam through sports physicals and sick visits until they became young adults. This ideal motivated me while I memorized structures of amino acids, innervation to each muscle in the human body, and learned the branches of the brachial plexus in pre-clinical studies. It is that picture of Sarah that I thought about every time I assisted in a baby's delivery or gave an Apgar score during medical school and pediatrics residency. I think of that picture now when I make nursery rounds and meet each new mom. Sarah reminds me that every life is precious.

Emily Vigour MD, FAAP
Pediatrician, Marrero, Louisiana

Preface

My daughter Sarah's birth on May 3, 1981, was one of the most joyous moments I have ever known. Her death, also on May 3, 1981, remains the most difficult loss I have ever had to come to terms with. That loss was additionally painful because most people I was in contact with after she died said things that were incongruous to what I was experiencing. Their reactions, without fault or blame, stemmed from a cultural lack of understanding of this particular death. It wasn't until the 1990s that the medical community began to believe that the deaths of newborns or stillborns were worthy of grief. (Surely women who miscarry and never have the babies they desperately want must suffer unimaginably. I was one of the lucky ones; although, I miscarried numerous times, I did, in the end, have three beautiful, healthy babies.) I trusted my reactions to Sarah's death because I had grieved before. My anguish after my brothers and my father's deaths had been validated. Yet Sarah's death, the most difficult one to deal with, was not – in most incidences – validated. She was my future. Books I read about newborn death didn't address the devastation, the catastrophic emotions I was experiencing. When I read that the death of a child is the most difficult one to accept, I began to get some support for my reactions. Then I read that the death of a child at any age: newborn to adult is the worst loss. One doesn't hurt less if the child is younger or hurt more if the child is older when he or she dies. Parents who have buried children, I read, would be in a trauma unit if their bodies were damaged as much as their psyches are after their child dies. That statement began to address the tidal-wave onslaught of the emotions I experienced after Sarah died.

I thought of my mother who was bereft after the deaths of her sons, Robert at seven months' gestation, and Little Joe who lived a year and a half. I don't think she ever recovered from those deaths and the lack of emotional support when she needed it most. She wasn't reacting as 'the experts' said she should. She was sad and experts told her to move on. I wanted to tell her story, as well as I know it, of what happens to unresolved grief. I wanted to show how it feels when a pregnancy ends in miscarriage or newborn death and a doctor or nurse says to have another baby. Experiencing, not squelching grief, is the only way to recover.

I also wanted to show as well as I could remember from the days, weeks and months after Robert and Little Joe died what it was like to be a child then, a forgotten mourner, and liken that memory to my own forgotten mourners, my daughters, Molly and Emily.

Childbirth has become medicalized out of fear of lawsuits and, I think, our increased knowledge of the process. I remember when my daughter, Emily, was in medical school, and she called to tell me that she had stripped a woman's membranes while she was in labor. I thought of the pain of someone's fingers separating the amniotic sack from the vaginal wall while in labor. Are we doing things in labor and delivery rooms because they are beneficial or because we know how to do them? The mother and her baby should be our first consideration. I would like to see more dignity in labor and delivery rooms and more respect for the natural process and the continuation of the love affairs that begin when two people want a baby.

Finally and most importantly, I wrote this book because babies are dying or being permanently injured in countries throughout the world because of group B streptococcus. With screening and treatment, the disease is preventable. As Sharon Hillier, PhD, the director of Reproductive Infectious Disease Research at Magee-Women's Hospital in Pittsburgh, Pennsylvania, says, 'Women need to be good healthcare consumers. They need to ask questions.'

I have changed the name of the neonatologist, and have given few details of our town, so that he and it are not recognizable. I realize that dialog cannot be remembered precisely from years ago. I ask the reader to suspend disbelief and imagine that the conversations might have occurred.

About the author

Theresa Huttlinger Vigour is a freelance writer, adjunct instructor of English, and a creative writing teacher. She has a bachelor's degree in journalism, a master's degree in English, and a master of fine arts degree in creative nonfiction writing.

Acknowledgements

Thanks to Janis Johnston and Sharon Williamson, my first readers, and Gillian Nineham, Editorial Director at Radcliffe Publishing, who believed in this book and to Ollie Judkins for his good humor and tireless editing. Thanks to my walking buddies, Cindy Morgan Baum and Lynn Barnes, who encouraged me year after year and mile after mile. Thanks to Molly and Emily who lived this story with their dad and me. And thanks to Kate for bringing hope back into our family. Finally, thanks to Tom who early on in our marriage wanted me to get a normal job and be a teacher or a nurse. When I told him that I couldn't be anything but a writer, he stopped hoping for normal and has been on this writing journey with me ever since.

Thanks to Randy S. Edelman, composer of *Weekend in New England*, for his lyrics.

·

PART 1

1. Anticipation

Sitting at a picnic table at the sailing club 11 days before the baby's due date, I dared not hope that he or she would come early or even on time. I estimated that I had a couple of weeks to wait as Molly had arrived four days after she was due and Emily four days earlier than she was expected. My longings for this baby had me acting out of character; I am seldom one to do anything ahead of time, more likely in the nick of time, but my overnight bag was already packed.

Advanced pregnancy either improved my hearing or I concentrated on sounds so I could sit longer. The sounds began at the farthest reaches of the pier that curved, tendril-like, and stretched a hundred feet into the river, one of several that are part of the intracoastal waterways of North Carolina. Untethered halyards tapped aluminum masts heralding offshore breezes while waves caressed sailboat hulls, as if they were made for each other. Seagulls glided and swooped over swirling waters created by the currents of brackish cove water mixing with the saltier river. Every few seconds a seagull trumpeted a battle cry before diving for a minnow. At the water's edge, tall marsh reeds swished percussion-like at the wind's command. The swish, the cries, waves lapping ceaselessly, halyards playing aluminum flutes were weekday sounds often overpowered on summer weekends by children's shrieks and giggles, sailors' laughter, boats being unloaded, cars pulling empty, clanging trailers, and the roar of outboard motors used to maneuver in and out of the harbor.

As afternoon turned to evening, the colors of the setting sun splashed ever-changing cascades of pinks, blues, purples, and lavenders. In contrast, the horizon became a black and white silhouette of loblolly pine trees whose branches and needles top the trees like an afterthought, the way mistletoe perches. Neither looks inherent. No skyscraper, no plant billowing smoke marred the view in this sparsely populated piece of land that juts into the Pamlico Sound.

Whenever the girls or scenes at the club or work would take my thoughts away from the new baby, I'd be jolted back to imagining holding him or her with intensified anticipation. A Braxton Hicks contraction, the involuntary tightening of the womb's muscles without any sensation of pain, or a baby kick would be enough to start the butterflies in my stomach, the it's-almost-Christmas feeling I'd get when I was ten. Getting pregnant and staying pregnant was not easy for me. After three miscarriages in three and a half years, I was on a high waiting for this baby's birth. Tom and I had been to infertility doctors and bared our souls as well as our body cavities and their contents. I cringed at the first question the urologist asked Tom, a nervous stutterer, 'Can you get it up?' I was relieved to hear his one-syllable response. I was the one who desperately wanted another child; I submitted to the questions, needles, blood tests, ovary squeezing, daily temperature readings and chartings, anything to get pregnant and stay pregnant. Eight months and three days earlier, for the fourth time in 30 months of trying, my morning body temperature remained elevated for more than two weeks, indicating fertilization.

For this baby, my mother found an antique cradle of warm walnut that rocked silently on metal hooks worn smooth. My mother had cut new foam padding for a mattress and hemmed miniature sheets. Tom's grandmother had made a multi-colored quilt of small squares for Molly's doll bed that just fit the cradle; Molly had loaned her quilt to the new baby. The cradle was next to my side of the bed.

The soft, yellow infant gown that my mother had sent before Molly was born was in the bag I'd packed for the hospital, as was the coral-colored gown, robe and slippers she had sent me before Emily's birth. The package had come days before Emily did. I opened it while sitting in the car parked outside the post office. The gown, edged in white lace, was modest enough for the hospital. And the bodice was complete with a buttoned opening for nursing. The matching robe had deep inset pockets, and the slippers were trimmed with the same lace. I cried over the beauty of the gown, right there in the car in front of the post office. Also packed in my bag was a dress my friend Lindy had loaned me. Although it was a maternity dress, its pleats either expanded or lay flat, so I could wear it when pregnant or in those early weeks after.

That evening at the riverbank, the setting sun's ever-lowering slant of light put the girls in the shadows. I could hear them splashing in the water, but I could no longer see them. I shifted my large body on the bench seat of the picnic table so that I could stand up and waddle to the shore to watch my girls. As I stood, I felt something warm and wet. Instead of going toward the water, I asked Tom to check on the girls, and I walked to the club bathhouse where I discovered the dampness was a slight bit of clear, clean-smelling amniotic fluid.

2. Uncharted waters

As I unloaded the cooler, putting the fruit salad and leftover ham sandwiches in the refrigerator, I called to the girls to pack their bags with clean shorts and a top each, undies, toothbrushes, jammies, and anything else they wanted to take to Grammie's house. I think the baby is coming tonight, I told them.

While Tom helped the girls gather teddy bears, toys, and, I hoped, clothes, I called my obstetrician at home and told him that a little amniotic fluid had leaked.

'It's too early for you to be in labor,' he said, but not in his normally attentive voice. Understandable, I thought, as he was at home where he might have been distracted by his four children or his wife who was expecting their fifth child in two weeks.

'It's just 11 days until my due date. My second baby was four days early.'

I expected him to say something like, 'pack a bag and meet me at the hospital,' but instead he said, 'It must be urine.'

'I know the difference.'

'You can meet me at the hospital, and I'll tell you it's urine.'

'I don't think that is necessary,' I told him before I said goodbye.

'What'd the doctor say?' Tom asked while carrying the girls' bags from their bedroom past the kitchen where I was.

'He said it's too early for labor to begin, so the leaking is urine.'

'But it's not, is it?'

'No.'

'What do we do now, T?' Tom asked

'I don't know, let me think out loud. The doctor didn't say to come to the hospital, and he didn't say not to come. He just said if we went, he'd tell me the wetness is urine. He didn't say what would happen if it's amniotic fluid. We could go to the hospital and see what happens. But the doctor was unconcerned so maybe he'd just send us home. It's almost nine. If we go to the hospital, it will be after midnight before we get home. We could just lie down for a while until contractions start. We could be in for a long night, and I really am tired.'

I showered and put on a clean maternity dress, one of my favorites because it was a bright mixture of plaids and patterns of flowers. The dress, another loan from Lindy whose husband, like Tom, was a forester at the paper company, drew attention to itself rather than to my ever-growing womb. I lay on top of the bedspread and smoothed out the folds of the dress, knowing that this would be the last time I would lie down with my womb full of baby. Three children were all Tom felt he could support emotionally and financially and I agreed, albeit reluctantly. Before Tom and I were married he'd talked about having four children, which had sounded good to me. By even thinking of a number, I was breaking away from the teachings of the Catholic church, the teachings that led to my mother's 14 pregnancies and eight live births and eventually led me to think that women must be more than breeders. I wanted a time after children to pursue a writing career. So I closed my eyes that night knowing contractions would start at any minute. When they did, it wouldn't be long before the baby would come, and I could lie on my stomach for the first time in six months.

I woke abruptly because the sun was shining. Last night was baby night, I thought. I heard Tom in the kitchen making coffee. Molly and Em were watching Captain Kangaroo on television.

'Well, sunshine, how are the contractions?' Tom bubbled with the banter of a morning person.

'No contractions.'

'Well, what now? I have to tell them something at the office.'

'I don't know. I've never had this happen before.'

'So this is a regular day then?'

I opened my mouth to speak, but I didn't have an answer. I didn't know the answer.

'In that case, I'm going to work,' he said businesslike.

Fire season in eastern North Carolina ran from Emily's birthday, February 27, to mine, May 18, which meant Tom missed both those birthdays and his own in March and countless family dinners and events in between, because he had to be on standby 24 hours a day, every day. Sometimes he could be on standby at home, but that season before our third child was born was drier than usual, so he and the other foresters had to go to the office on Saturdays or be out checking hot spots.

Tom is a scientist both in his genes and in his education and training. He approaches situations unemotionally as he would a math calculation. He wanted a yes or no answer rather than a maybe or an I don't know. He understood my reluctance to go to the hospital and knew, as I did, that submitting to procedures unnecessary for a normal birth more often than not causes problems. He knew I'd go when active labor began but not before I had to. But Tom defers to facts, to authority, and leaking amniotic fluid, though slight and intermittent, was a sign that labor had begun. His confidence and self-assuredness, the qualities I, an introvert, fell in love with, are the same traits that make him overbearing when I don't agree with him.

'Do you know where you'll be today?'

'Not really. Fires are breaking out all over. But if you need me, call Penny. She'll know where I am,' he said, putting a leftover ham sandwich into his lunch box.

A sandwich in his lunch box. He's putting a ham sandwich into his lunch box. He really is going to leave for work. There are no gray areas in his life. I wished he'd stay home and spend some time with me in my gray area, which was in between knowing that healthy babies can be born weeks after membranes rupture and the fact that contractions could start the minute he pulled his truck out of the driveway. If they did, in those pre-cell-phone days, there was time for him to drive the 40 minutes to work, get my message and drive home, get me, and drive to the hospital another 45 minutes away. Tom would be taking a day or two off work to be with me during labor and delivery; 12-week maternity leaves, paid or unpaid, for mothers and fathers were not in place in 1981. So he had to be sure that labor had begun before he began his leave.

Tom had taken the top off the empty cookie canister and was looking inside.

'There is an unopened bag of cookies in the cabinet,' I told him.

When Tom got to work, I later learned, he mentioned to one of the secretaries that my water had broken. He didn't say the membranes oozed occasionally, creating dampness like perspiration; he said the water had broken. Naturally, the secretary said that I should be in a hospital. An older woman who had had a baby represented an authority figure to him.

T can be hard-headed, Tom thought. She ought to listen more to doctors. Yes, they've done things to her in hospitals that I wouldn't want done to me, and she's had to fight both nurses and doctors to be able to nurse the babies, but we had two healthy kids. That's the bottom line.

He called my obstetrician.

I drove with the girls to my mother's house. Her guest bed was so snuggle-into soft that I felt hugged and grateful to be tired. I slept until she knocked at the door, 'Phone for you.'

'Theresa,' the obstetrician said, 'your husband called me. He told me I might reach you here. So, your water broke.'

'Last night you said it was urine,' I reminded him.

'After membranes have been ruptured more than 24 hours, there is a risk of infection.'

'I don't want to be induced. I'm afraid to speed up labor – that might create problems.'

'I won't do anything you don't want me to do,' he said before saying goodbye.

I tried to put the receiver back on the hook, but it slipped. My hand was shaking. The obstetrician said he would allow labor to progress naturally, that he wouldn't interfere, but would he? The doctor that I used for Emily's birth said he would not interfere with the natural process, but when labor started he intervened both medically and surgically.

3. Tradition, technology and the women's movement

When I was pregnant for the first time in 1974 – after years of trying – I hadn't intended to make a study of labor and delivery until a neighbor whom I knew only by sight told me that having a baby is torture. 'The pain is like nothing you can imagine. Think of the worst toothache you've ever had and having a baby is worse than that.'

'That's before you get to the hospital. Then they give you something for pain, right?'

'Oh, boy, have you got a lot to learn. They don't give you any medicine for pain until you go to the delivery room.'

'How long is it before you go to the delivery room?'

'It can take days.'

My mother had talked about how quickly she forgot about labor when she held each new baby. 'Pain is its own anesthesia,' she'd say. Never had I heard anyone describe childbirth as torture.

A week later the neighbor came to visit, and, this time, she brought her husband. They sat Tom and me down and described the birth process as one pain after another, complete with details. The doctor had blood up to his elbows; it was amazing that nobody dropped the baby or slipped and fell on that blood-covered floor. Their descriptions included obscenities hurled at their boyfriends or husbands by otherwise controlled women.

'You'll lie there screaming or moaning for hours and hours all by yourself,' my neighbor continued.

After they left, Tom commented that it sounded like some rite of passage. 'You have to suffer to be a true woman,' he said wrapping his arms around his stomach. 'Damn you, Paul,' he mimicked the neighbor. His attempts to pacify my fears with humor didn't work. I called my friends Kath and Glenda who already had children.

'She may have exaggerated somewhat,' Kath said, 'but basically, yes, there's a lot of pain.'

'You can hurt just as much with a bad case of the flu,' Glenda said, 'and when it's over, what do you get? Nothing. After childbirth, you get a baby. It's worth it.'

I tried to push thoughts of childbirth pain to the back of my mind, as Molly's birth was months away. But my neighbors' stories and Kath's and Glenda's confirmation nagged at me. I am not stoic. I opt for nitrous oxide to open my mouth for my dentist.

In an effort to find a drug or some way to alleviate pain until the time of delivery, I asked other new mothers how they managed childbirth and began reading everything I could find on the subject. My cousin Beth from California told me she had had her baby without any pain medicine. 'You can take control and deliver your baby rather than be delivered of it,' she told me. 'It's better for you and your baby, but you've got to prepare. It's the hardest job we do. That's why they call it labor.' She was upbeat about the whole experience, unlike any other mother I'd talked to. She followed the Lamaze method detailed in *Thank You, Dr Lamaze* by Marjorie Karmel. She was so positive, so exhilarated, that I was fascinated. Each generation has its 'new' way of having babies: natural childbirth, childbirth without fear, twilight sleep, all with new methods of pain relief. Before Molly's birth in the era that ushered in hippies, birth control, and Women's Liberation, natural childbirth – Lamaze – was the method of choice among educated women, and its popularity flourished, but mostly in the more populated regions.

Karmel described the method that she learned in France: *accouchement sans douleur* or childbirth without pain. I thought that if I had to wait for days until I could have something for pain, I could use this method for the unmedicated part of labor. As I practiced the mental and physical exercises in the book, I began to trust in the natural birth process and gained confidence in myself and in my ability to manage labor without drugs. I read that almost any drug would cross the placenta and adversely affect the baby. Without drugs, both mother and baby are most alert in the hours just after birth. Babies will not be that alert until weeks later – another one of nature's gifts: time to say hello.

Tom liked the idea of being my labor coach and was enthusiastic about the training: he'd time practice contractions and encourage me to keep going. Ever the keeper of records, ever the scientist, Tom bought a new stopwatch and kept a pad of paper in his pocket in the last weeks of pregnancy to record contractions. Noting the strength and duration would track labor's progress. As he grew into his new role, I found myself becoming more and more comforted knowing he would be with me and would have some knowledge of what I was experiencing. I would not labor alone.

A more deep-seated reason Lamaze appealed to me was the opportunity to see the baby right after it was born, to learn its sex and if it was all right; alert, I could do something if it wasn't. My mother told of waking up after the anesthesia from childbirth wore off to learn that her fifth child, my brother Robert, had died; she was the last one in the hospital and in our family to hear the news. Her doctor thought that mom's flu and continuous coughing caused his arrival two months prematurely. He died of a breathing problem particular to preemies, hyaline membrane disease, now known as respiratory distress syndrome. He was in the morgue by the time she woke up; she never saw him.

Although Karmel's book was originally published in 1959, and classes in the Lamaze method of childbirth were available on the West Coast and in large cities, the method was unheard of by many people in rural areas in the 1970s. What I came to realize was that I was studying the French method of *laissez faire* childbirth, but I would be under the care of American doctors who are trained to medically manage labor with drugs, machines, and scalpels. Further, three opposing forces were operating at once in the labor and delivery rooms during the mid-1970s and early 1980s: tradition, technology, and the women's movement.

Traditionally, women were given medicine so that they could not feel or remember much about childbirth. It was an era of: trust me, I'm the doctor. The women my neighbor told me about who shouted obscenities at their babies' fathers were not reacting to a normal part of the birth process; they were drug-crazed. Even if they didn't remember the obscenities, their husbands did.

Technology was developing and being used more and more to electronically monitor the mother's contractions and the baby's heartbeats. The oft-repeated words – *this procedure is necessary to ensure the safety of your baby* – was turning out to have the opposite effect. The rate of Caesarean births was skyrocketing to half of all births in some hospitals as the new technology spit out reams of printouts of the mother's contractions and baby's heartbeats during labor and delivery. Often stress was read as distress and emergency Caesarean sections were performed. The new monitors made it necessary for mothers to recline and remain still, so heartbeats and contractions could be recorded without interference. That position is not only uncomfortable to maintain throughout labor, it puts pressure on the artery supplying the placenta with oxygen and nutrients. Sonograms were beginning to be used to diagnose abnormalities, look for multiple births, and determine the baby's sex. IVs during labor were coming into use. 'Just in case something goes wrong, we have a line available.'

The women's movement had entered the labor and delivery rooms in large cities, though not in rural areas, so women were beginning to believe that they had some say about what was being done to their bodies. These forces combined to create confusion and frustration for pregnant women and their healthcare providers. Agendas conflicted. Fear and loss of power abounded about a normal process that is, 95% of the time, uneventful.

Molly's 12-hour labor was normal and manageable with the exercises I'd practiced from Karmel's book. The only odd thing that happened was when a nurse handed Molly to me, and she was wrapped in paper stiff as a brown grocery bag. The nurse said I'd break the germ field if I touched her. So, Molly nursed on the delivery table while I stroked her through the stiff blue paper. I guess my arms and hands were germy but my nipples were not. I was too happy to question the nurse. It was then, in the moments after Molly's birth, that I understood my cousin Beth's exhilaration. The emotional high was like nothing else I'd ever experienced; drugged, I would have missed that joy.

My obstetrician was overloaded with patients when I was pregnant with Emily a year later, in 1975, so I looked for another. Three other doctors in the area delivered babies. Two obstetricians were not receptive to Lamaze, the other doctor was a family practitioner, probably in his 60s, neat, proper, subdued. He agreed to my using the Lamaze method, which turned out to mean little because he and the rural hospital staff were not familiar with natural childbirth.

All my pubic hair was shaved before Emily's birth. Telling the nurses that I'd prefer they not do it and that I'd already had a baby without the shaving did not stop them. 'This prevents infection,' a nurse told me. 'Doctor's orders.' For weeks my crotch was itchy, prickly, and infected with pimply ingrown hairs. I read later that shaving pubic hair before birth is as necessary to preventing infection as is removing a man's mustache and beard before extracting a tooth.

The doctor ruptured my membranes during his first examination after I came to the hospital in labor, eliminating the natural cushion for the baby's head and brain as it was pushed against the pelvic bones during contractions. He then had a nurse give me Pitocin, a drug used to speed up labor. I told the nurse that my first labor progressed without drugs. I was afraid of an artificially speeded up labor because my friend Carol's brother died during childbirth. Her mother was having her third child during wartime in England. The doctor was overworked and in a hurry, so he gave her drugs to make her labor go faster. My friend's mother begged not to be given the drugs, telling the doctor and the nurses that her past labors had only lasted a couple of hours. The baby died of a brain hemorrhage because he was born too quickly.

The doctor also ordered that my legs be strapped down on the delivery table. Being strapped down while every inch of my body was working to push the baby was dehumanizing. The use of stirrups for delivery, I had read, began not for the mother's convenience but so a husband could have a better view of his child's birth. Being strapped to stirrups in a flat position during labor made as much sense as assuming that position for urination or defecation. The doctor cut through my perineum rather than let the baby slip through the soft tissue. It was my first and only episiotomy.

'Stop breathing like that. You'll hyperventilate,' a labor room nurse yelled a hundred times while I was pushing Emily. It took an enormous amount of concentration to continue to tune her out. After I delivered Emily, she asked me how I had the baby without anesthesia. She sounded genuinely curious.

'By breathing the way I did,' I told her.

Emily lay in an isolet, a clear plastic bin about twice the size of a shoebox. The container is aptly named; she was isolated. Her eyes were big and searching as she gazed around the room. She looked so small and lonely.

'Please let me hold her,' I begged.

'Of course not,' the nurse said with all the force she used to try to keep me from breathing.

As the doctor was stitching the incision back together, he told me he was taking a few extra stitches for my husband. Today that remark would be labeled sexist and reprimands would be imminent. But then I lay there – with my legs tied down with leather straps while being stitched back together following surgery that I specifically said I did not want – a slave to modern medicine. I learned that the wounds of indignity last for lifetimes. I was never able to use tampons after that episiotomy; the scar tissue prevented the muscles from contracting normally, and the tampons fell out.

I was not allowed to hold, feed or see Emily for another 24 hours as the nurses told me that she would be drinking water until my milk came in. The colostrum, made for infants' first feedings, and dubbed 'liquid gold' for all the nutrients and antibodies it contains, was reabsorbed into my system. Emily and I were both victims.

Veterinarians, cattle breeders, and pet owners do not prevent their new-mother animals from nuzzling, licking, or nursing their newborns. Animal mothers were treated with more respect than human mothers. Emily, who was not held by anyone until hours after she was born, became our only child to suffer painfully from homesickness, and I've often wondered if the isolation of those first hours and during her first day of life is the reason.

I thought about the importance of holding newborns when my veterinarian friend and I were comparing our two cats, one who craved attention, the other who tolerated people. A bonding takes place, Jan said. Holding, stroking, and petting newborn kittens almost always ensures that they will be affectionate pets. I used to think that the breed of cat determined its loving or aloof nature. Siamese cats, I thought, were born to be as mean as my friend Abby's Siamese, Honeycomb, who would perch on the top of a door frame and drop onto our heads as we'd pass under him. Yet early handling breeds trust in all kinds of cats: Siamese, Himalayan, Tabby, alley cats. You don't make up later for the lack of handling of kittens in the early days and weeks after birth, Jan said.

Soon after Emily was taken to the nursery and I was wheeled to my room, a nurse announced that she was going to catheterize me. I told her I did not need a catheter to aid urination because I had had my baby without anesthesia. She was adamant. I told her I would like to talk to my doctor. She said she was not leaving the room until I was catheterized. I am a strong person. I know my rights. Yet, less than an hour after delivery, and after the sleep-deprived nights in the last weeks of pregnancy, and lying in bed in a hospital gown, I was not coming from my usual position of strength. I relented, feeling as if I had been raped by that nurse. She was so angry at not being able to extract any urine from my bladder that she leaned on my stomach until I thought she would squeeze my uterus out of the weakened vaginal walls. She never got a drop. I was determined that for the next baby, I would find an obstetrician or a midwife who understood natural childbirth.

Dates and charts became an obsession when infertility persisted for so long that I began measuring it in years. My focus was on the 48 hours or less during each month when conception could occur – the time after the ovary releases an egg. I maximized my chances of conceiving by knowing when those 48 hours were by taking my temperature each morning and making graphs. A rise in temperature would indicate ovulation and intercourse could be timed accordingly. For the first year that I took my temperature, trying to conceive for the first time, my graphs showed straight lines, no temperature change, no ovulation, no possibility of conception. My obstetrician prescribed synthroid to regulate my body clock so it would operate at the proper speed and produce the proper amounts of hormones to initiate ovulation. It worked. I didn't conceive for another 14 months, but the rise in temperature each month gave me hope. Molly's pregnancy was followed quickly by Emily's. When Emily was two we began trying to have another baby. In a few months, I was happily pregnant. Weeks later, I miscarried – a spontaneous abortion, medical books call it. Twice more I was pregnant and miscarried early.

I had temperature charts, dates of ovulation, and times of optimum fertility down to a science by the time my graphs showed a victorious rise in temperature indicating the conception of our third child, two and a half years in the making. The date of conception was August 27, the day my grandmother died and the same month and day as her son's, my father's death, 16 years earlier. A sign? The heavens smiling. A continuum. Death and birth. Sadness and joy.

As the pregnancy progressed, I started focusing on the birth, specifically a home birth. No stirrups, no straps, no catheters, no shaving, no nurse to yell at me, no one to tell me I couldn't hold my baby. My friend Anne, a nurse, said she really wished she could help me with a home birth, but if she did, she wouldn't ever be able to work in a hospital again. It's frowned upon by doctors, she told me. 'I'd be blackballed,' she said. Her words were echoed by other nurses, and no midwives practiced on their own in our area. So I would have to go to a hospital to have the third baby. My apprehension was building as it was becoming difficult to trust doctors who would agree to things in the office and then, in the hospital, they would do what they wanted. I'd read, though, that women could claim some power by laboring at home before going to the hospital. That way, doctors and nurses would have less time to hook them up to machines and give drugs.

My brother Carl's girlfriend mentioned her obstetrician/gynecologist who practiced in a small town 45 minutes away. 'I think you'd like him,' she said. He was all for prepared childbirth.

He even had a nurse-midwife help him sometimes with hospital deliveries. He was a kind man, young.

'I want to hold the baby after it's born,' I told the doctor the day I met him.

'That's fine with me,' he said.

'If the baby wants to nurse right away, I'd like to let it.'

'My wife has nursed all our babies on the delivery table.'

'I don't want stirrups, or my arms or legs strapped down and no episiotomy.'

'You do sound like my wife. She doesn't care for them either. I see no need for stirrups or strapping.'

So I began seeing this obstetrician.

Toward the end of the pregnancy, he mentioned that my delivery would be monitored electronically with external and internal monitors. I'd read what was happening in labor and delivery rooms: medical technology had added even more equipment since Emily's birth. For at-risk pregnancies, the new technology was saving the lives of babies who otherwise might not have survived. But for the majority of pregnancies the new technology was causing problems and inconveniencies to mothers who wanted labor to progress naturally.

Electronic monitors are more precise than the human ear, my doctor said. With them, we can record all the heartbeats since the monitors stay in place throughout labor and delivery. That way we can know how the baby's heart is functioning throughout labor.

I told him that I couldn't manage labor contractions with a strap around my stomach. And that if I could walk and change positions that my labor would progress more quickly. If I could manage labor contractions, then I wouldn't need drugs and that would be good for the baby. Is an external monitor necessary? I asked him. I've never had one before. Do you anticipate problems with this delivery?

No, he didn't expect any problems, but added that an external monitor provides information. And internal monitors can detect heart defects and the strength of contractions.

I knew that the internal monitor was screwed into the baby's scalp, and through that electrode, nurses and doctors could hear the baby's heartbeat. I had read that babies with internal monitors are more likely to be born by Caesarean section since the monitors transmit more information.

'Do we need this information?' I asked the doctor. 'Especially if it's an inconvenience to me and might be enough of an inconvenience that I'd need drugs?'

'Probably not,' he said at a negotiating session. 'I'll give you an IV for no internal monitor.'

I agreed. At least I would get stuck and not the baby.

Those conversations had taken place weeks earlier at the doctor's office. We'd rehearsed many scenarios, but not what we would do if the membranes oozed. So there I was at my mother's house, not sure what to do, when I heard a knock at her front door.

4. She's perfect

My mother answered the kitchen door that opened from the garage, and I heard Tom's voice before I saw him. 'T, did the doctor call? What did he say?'

'That after 24 hours there's a risk of infection.'

'And?'

'I told the doctor I wanted to wait for contractions to start.'

'What did he say to that?' Tom asked.

'Goodbye.'

'Well, if everybody is happy, I'm going back to work,' Tom said.

'If you're going back to work, then you won't be here to help me.'

'What help do you need?' he asked standing on one foot, then the other, growing increasingly agitated.

I wanted him to be gentle with me, to step out of his character, his analytical, just-the-facts self and put his arms around me and let me feel safe, protected. But he's neither a mind reader, nor is he able to read between the lines of people's emotions, not even mine. In the early years of our marriage, when his insensitivity clashed with my hypersensitivity, I cried or sulked. Later, I tried to develop a thicker skin and not take his wry, humorous, or sarcastic comments as insults to my cooking or decorating or house cleaning. And I learned to retort. Sometimes, he'd respond with *touché* or *ouch*, feeling the sting his words could deliver.

His jokes were funny to him when I was the brunt, but not so when he was. Even when his comments seem unromantic or thoughtless, he is honest, and though I've had to set limits – do not tell me I look fat and do not compare my cooking to your mother's – I am more grateful than not for his honesty. Sarcastic though he is, I always know where I stand with Tom, unlike with my mother, who would not speak to us children or our dad for days, rather than say what was bothering her. Growing up I felt managed by her silences, as I'd try to figure out how I'd hurt her feelings. I appreciate Tom's directness even when it stings. That sting, signifying our personality differences, is minor, really, in a marriage that is supportive. But when the stakes were higher, our differences were paramount. His increasing impatience at my unwillingness to go to the hospital before contractions started grew like a wall between us. Yet we were working toward the same end, and I knew when active labor began, he would be there for me – coaching and encouraging – just as steady and sure as he is.

'I don't need help,' I told him. 'Just go on.'

I thanked Mom for watching the girls while I napped, and we headed for home for lunch. I took the curvy road by the country club. The asphalt is a deep, dark, stunning black – stunning next to the emerald-green golf course. When I drive this again, I thought, I'll have the new baby.

Molly, Em, and I ate peanut butter sandwiches with home-made strawberry preserves. Together we collected dirty laundry from the bedrooms, sorted, washed, dried, and folded clothes. We picked up toys from the living room and kitchen floors. When the girls grew tired of helping and stopped to play by themselves, I could do things I needed to do by myself like sort through the afternoon's mail while I listened to them. Molly kept the tempo, the energy level, ratcheted up. She is a motion machine, happiest when she has something to do, learn, or explore. She is exhilarating. In contrast, Emily could play with her dolls for hours with or without a friend. If Molly was quiet I worried that she was sick or doing something she didn't want me to know. If Emily was noisy, I became concerned. Soon it was time to cook dinner. The afternoon had gone by so fast that I didn't have time to think about the slight bit of amniotic fluid that continued to dampen pads, but only when I walked, not when I stood still or sat.

Late in the afternoon, the obstetrician's nurse-midwife called to say that she was on duty that night, and she didn't want to be delivering my baby after midnight. She was an abrupt woman with the clipped, no-nonsense, don't-mess-with-me tone I'd heard from New Yorkers when visiting my grandparents in Manhattan. She didn't ask me anything; she just made the statement and hung up.

After dinner, I went for a walk mostly to have a little time alone, emotional-battery-charging time for an introvert. I walked gently with my heavy loads of baby, eagerness, and fears. I walked in the middle of our quiet street paved with stones that reminded me of the cobblestone street near where I grew up in historic Alexandria, Virginia. I walked two houses away, just past Glennie Rhodes' house, when a contraction immobilized me. I never did learn to call her Glennie although she had asked me to many times. My sweet friend, who was old enough to be my grandmother, had helped three-year-old Molly plant pansies in a part of our side yard that she could see from her front porch. We laughed the next day when Molly watered her pansies in the rain. She wore her yellow plastic raincoat with matching hat and tipped the blue flowered watering can that the Easter Bunny had given her just weeks before.

'Call me Glennie,' she'd say in the first years we lived next door.

'Have I no respect for my neighbor's white hair?' I'd ask.

'But, please, nearly all my friends are dead. If you call me Glennie rather than Mrs Rhodes, then I have another friend alive.'

I was too young then to know what she meant. I was someone's granddaughter then. I should have called her Glennie for her sake and my own regrets later.

A contraction started then, just past Mrs Rhodes' house and before DE Smythe's house. I don't remember ever seeing him or hearing the neighbors talk about him. He grew a tall cane barrier between his yard and the street. The neighbors appreciated individuals and their quirks as they do in old, settled streets like ours. So in the middle of our quiet street beside DE Smythe's house, I was unable to move. It's strange how short two minutes are when you're walking and trying to get home before the next contraction starts. And it's strange how long a 45-second contraction is when you are immobilized by its strength. I walked, stopped, walked, stopped, stopped, stopped. It was 20 minutes before I got back to the house.

'This is it,' I grinned after finally making it to the front porch, where Tom was smoking a cigar and Molly and Emily were trying to catch early summer fireflies. 'We've got contractions.'

All the fire drills were over. Tom, Molly, Emily grabbed bags, books, teddy bears, toothbrushes, suitcases, pillows, sandwiches, called Grammie, called bosses. I sat and breathed and timed contractions and felt connected to generations of women by this painful, natural, normal passage in progress. When you want a baby, life moves eternally slowly for nine months like a leaf floating on a meandering creek. It seems to be going nowhere until a narrow shoot appears and the elevation drops. Suddenly the trickle becomes a gush, and the leaf is propelled through the channel and into the main stream.

Tom drove us to my mother's house where we left Molly and Emily and exchanged quick kisses and hugs. My youngest brother Pete said, 'They'll have ice cream, cookies, gum, candy every day, all day,' teasing me about our house rules of limiting sweets.

'Don't you dare,' I cautioned the college freshman who was laughing too hard to hear me.

'See you, T,' he said, and waved and grinned. I'd carried him for years before his heart surgery. His weak heart would not allow him to walk very far, so I carried him piggyback for five years until I started college. The doctors didn't think he'd live. A prognosis like that makes all of us appreciate the time we spend with him.

'See you,' I called from my front passenger seat in the car. Such a little goodbye. How to say more and breathe too?

'It's happnin',' my brother Carl said.

'You've got it, bro. It's happnin',' I told him.

Then Tom and I were alone and he said, 'Why didn't you do what the doctor told you and go to the hospital this morning when he called you?'

'He didn't tell me to go to the hospital,' I said while looking at my watch to see how much time I had before I would be motionless and speechless and focusing on the self-hypnotic pain management during another contraction. I was the one facing labor and delivery and scared of what would be done to me and knowing what little control I would have once I entered the hospital.

'But your water broke,' he said. 'Shouldn't you have been doing something?'

'Correction: oozed slightly, occasionally. I did do something. I called the doctor right away. I figured he'd say to come to the hospital. I figured labor had started. But when he wasn't concerned, I tried not to be. Anyway, I was doing something. You got to go to work, have a regular, A-okay day while I'm at home wondering what is happening.'

'Damn it, do you have to be so hard-headed? I don't want a dead baby.'

'You're angry because I didn't go to the hospital right away, didn't do what you wanted, didn't do it your way. Now that we're going to the hospital, now that I'm trying my best to manage contractions, you're swearing at me.'

Yes he was angry, but in retrospect, scared was coming out angry. I had contractions to keep my mind off a slight bit of fluid seeping and all my hopes that this wasn't a bad sign and all my fears that it was.

'Do we have a name yet for this baby?' Tom asked, changing the subject.

Tom can pick out the new baby's name early on in the pregnancy, and once he has, he is content with his decision. I agonize over names. Will playmates invent hurtful nicknames based upon our choices? Have we adequately represented both sides of the family? Only once did my mother mention a baby name to me. 'Have you thought about Joe?' Joseph Bernard Huttlinger was my father's name.

'I can't, Mom,' I told her. 'It's unlucky.' We'd had three Joes die in our family. She understood. For each baby, Tom and I discussed baby names up until signing the birth certificates. Although he becomes annoyed with my indecision, mostly the exchanges are upbeat, as we look forward to the new baby. But on the way to the hospital that evening, we were not in our usual upbeat pick-a-name moods.

'Josh, if it's a boy. But if it's a girl, I don't know.'

'Laura. It's always been Laura. What are you saying, "You don't know." My God, for years we've talked about Laura as a baby's name. What's your problem? Sometimes, no, a lot of times, I don't know where you are coming from. You have lots of information, you read all the time and yet you do something stupid like not going to the hospital when your water breaks.'

'Are you ever going to let up? Now you call me stupid. Here I am trying to have a baby. Not fun. Not my idea of an ideal Saturday night. There are plenty of other things I can think of that I would like to be doing now rather than having contractions. It is biologically impossible for you to know what I am experiencing right now, but I can assure you this is not the time to berate me, criticize me, or fight with me. And if a contraction weren't starting, I would tell you that I have never liked the name Laura – never, ever. That name was in your head, in your imagination, you never cleared it with me. And now, when I'm having a baby, you lay it on me that you have always assumed that if we had a girl, she would be named Laura.'

Laura. I never could figure out how to pronounce Laura: Loura or Lawra or Lalra. And I didn't much care for the sounds I made every time I practiced saying the name. Occasionally, when other people said the name, it sounded beautiful, as when Omar Sharif in *Dr Zhivago* called to his love, Lara. The sound of her name, said with the yearning of a secret lover, was the sound of adoration and desire matched only by Julie Christie's beauty. But I couldn't make Laura sound like anything I liked hearing.

'All right, then, Sarah,' Tom said.

Sarah? Sarah sounds Jewish and biblical. I'm Catholic. I'm not old-fashioned enough to use a 2000-year-old name, and I'm not that biblically inclined. Another contraction started. At least he wasn't still holding out for Laura.

'Okay, Sarah,' I said.

I was breathing in two-four time, to the tune of *Yankee Doodle*.

Contractions were two minutes apart and manageable when we arrived at the hospital at 9.00 p.m. I was using only slow chest breathing, saving the effleurage and superficial or accelerated breathing for later. I was not afraid of this baby's labor or delivery, but I was afraid of hospital procedures.

By 10.00 p.m., an IV had been inserted into a vein in the back of my left hand, making effleurage difficult. Effleurage, the gentle, feather-like motions made by the finger tips rhythmically stroking the lower stomach, helped relax those muscles and gave me something besides contractions to concentrate on. Effleurage is both physical and mental and part of the Lamaze method. It works for me, but this was the first time I had had an IV during labor. The IV dripped so much fluid into my veins that I needed to use the bathroom several times. The bathroom trips were distracting to the concentration necessary for managing labor.

Tom timed contractions and told me I was doing great. His voice was reassuring, calm, authoritative. I would have been lonely and scared without him, especially when the nurses left the room.

After midnight, the contractions gained in strength and duration. If this labor followed those of Molly's and Emily's, I would have an urge to push soon. Unexpectedly, my obstetrician was at the foot of my bed and equally as unexpected, he was dressed in a tuxedo. Did I want him to stay, he asked. I thought that he shouldn't miss a formal party for a delivery, not realizing, in my self-absorbed state, that the party was probably over. A nurse came to the door and asked if she and her friends could come and watch. I told her I didn't care and I didn't then; I didn't care about anything, as I must have been getting close to the mentally disorienting contractions of transition. The obstetrician left and nurses came in lining every inch of the walls of the delivery room. If I ever saw a woman in the last stages of labor, I promised myself that night that the only things I would ask her are, 'How can I help?' or 'What can I do to make you more comfortable?' Not, 'Can my friends and I watch?' I felt like a sideshow in a cheap traveling carnival. Or worse, since I was exposing all.

Then something happened. Unlike previous labors, unlike any contraction I had experienced, the pain became so severe that I blacked out. From sometime after midnight until nearly 3.00 a.m., I writhed. Once I regained consciousness to find myself on my knees facing the mattress. My arms were gripping metal support pieces of the bed frame; I bent them.

'Please do something,' I begged the nurse-midwife.

'No,' she responded.

I could see Tom's face; it showed no alarm. Not the alarm I would have expected if I were truly ripping apart as I felt I was.

I cried and blacked out again. Years later, I would learn the cause of the abnormal pain.

I woke up urinating in the bed I would deliver in. Damn IV – an opportunity for infection for the baby.

'Push,' the nurse-midwife yelled.

'I can see the head,' Tom said. With Molly's and Emily's deliveries, Tom had called out that he could see the baby's head and the excitement in his voice carried me from weariness to pushing, from wanting to go home, to finishing the job. With Molly and Emily, pushing had been a release. I had felt pressure, but no pain. But for the third delivery, the pain was unbearable. I was on fire. Tom's voice must have helped with that birth, too, because the next thing I heard was the nurse-midwife say, 'She's perfect.' Her perfect 10 was her Apgar Score which rates newborns according to activity, pulse, grimace, appearance, and respiration. Sarah scored two points on each, earning the highest possible, 10. Yet, Tom made a note in his diary later that day that Sarah was panting, breathing faster and more shallow after her birth than had Molly or Em.

I did not look at Sarah. I turned my head toward a blank space on a wall where there were no nurses, no onlookers, no babies, no IV stands, no monitors. I stared at the blank wall and closed my ears to the nurses' voices. Voices that had yelled became mumblings and my fiery pain burnt into memory. A nurse offered me a tiny oblong bundle no bigger than a large eggplant covered with a blanket of faded yellow and blue bunnies. I nodded. She tucked the bundle between my left arm and my side. How could one so small have caused so much pain? She was just 6 lbs and 1 oz, her head no bigger than an orange.

Sarah she was, the miracle in my arms. The longer I held her, the more I forgot about the painful delivery and the better she felt in my arms. I stroked her cheek, feather-like, and the skin on her forehead responded by wrinkling. Her damp hair looked black until I lifted strands, and the bright lights of the delivery room illuminated red hair. I could hear my mother when she would see Sarah's hair. 'The Lord has surely blessed us, T, with a red-haired baby.' My red-headed mother had eight brown-haired children. Sarah's eyes, rimmed in blue, opened wide in wonder, but no wider than mine as I gazed at the wonder of her.

Sarah's lips were outlined delicately as if by a tiny pink pencil. Her fingernails already needed cutting. Her curly black eyelashes highlighted her slate-blue eyes. Her wrinkly forehead skin that seemed loosely attached would become integral in just days. She whimpered and nuzzled, rubbing her cheek on my breast until she found the nipple. She held it securely with her gums and her redbud-pink lips and closed her eyes.

My body, which I had surrendered to passion and pregnancy, was now Sarah's. My breasts would fill with milk to accommodate her hunger and her need for comfort. Her needs would become mine. Her cry, even the sight of her, would cause my breasts to ache – an ache born of love and a need to give it away. Sarah Bancroft Vigour. Bancroft out of admiration for my great-grandmother who was ambitious and independent and the second woman to graduate from medical school in California.

The nurse-midwife took a picture of Sarah, who had fallen asleep with the nipple in her mouth. She caught my face in the picture looking more than happy, more like awe.

5. A slight breathing problem

Tom left the recovery room saying he would find us something to eat and meet me in my hospital room after a nurse announced, 'It's time,' and took Sarah from my arms. I watched Sarah until she left the room. Then I followed her in my mind as I imagined her being bathed and dressed and pricked with needles for blood tests. I imagined her getting eye drops to prevent blindness in case I had gonorrhea. Fair-skinned Molly and Emily had worn raccoon-like masks of irritation after nurses put drops in their eyes and the excess spilled out. For each of my babies I had asked that the drops not be put in their eyes as they irritate their skin, and I don't have gonorrhea. But the drops were put in as the law requires. So, the next time I saw Sarah, she would wear the mask of a hospital routine.

'Try and get some sleep, dear,' a delivery room nurse was saying as she wheeled a stretcher next to the delivery room bed. 'Here, now, scoot onto this stretcher, and I'll wheel you to your room so you can rest. You must be exhausted. You've been in labor how long? When did contractions start?'

'At 7.00,' I told her.

'Child, it's time to sleep. Come on now, ease on over a little more. That's it. Good,' she said, snapping the side rail into place and swinging the stretcher away from the delivery room bed.

'How many babies are in the nursery?' I asked as she wheeled me out of the delivery room.

'It's quiet tonight. Only two.'

Good. The nurses will have time to take good care of Sarah.

'When may I have my baby back?'

'Let's see, it's 5.00 a.m. On Sunday mornings the neonatologist doesn't check babies until about 9.00. So, say 9.30 a nursery nurse will bring her to you.'

'Here's your bed. Now scoot off this stretcher. And remember, call me if you want to get out of bed to shower or use the bathroom or whatever. Sleep now. There won't be much time to rest when you get that youngin' home.'

Rest. Rest? Does a sailor who has just won a race rest? She wants to shout for joy or hug friends and relatives. The moment is hers. After all the preparation, the pay back is exhilaration. It's champagne time. She moves as if doing calisthenics because joy is energizing. No one says, *time to rest*. On election night, does a president-elect feel like sleeping because some campaign organizer says, 'You'll have a big job to do come January. You'd better get some sleep, Mr President-elect.' He whoops and shouts. I did it. I won. The polls said we wouldn't win. It's time to relive each climb. Who would have thought we'd win in Illinois? Sleep? Now? Impossible.

I needed Sarah. After years of wanting her, I needed to hold her. Separation was unnatural. Had I had drugs for pain or fear of pain, I might have been drowsy or disoriented or groggy or unconscious, but I wasn't. I was high. I wanted to whisper softly in her ear: Hello, baby Sarah, you're mine. I'm here for you for always. You're part of a family who adores you. I wanted to watch Tom's face as he held her. I wanted to tell her about her dad, her sisters, her uncles, her cousins, her grandparents. I wanted to sing a love song. She knew my voice; she'd been hearing it for nine months. I wanted to memorize her yawns and stretches and study her soft new skin for characteristics of generations of my family and Tom's. Without her, piano music played in my mind as crisply as if the instrument and the player were in the room. I didn't will it; it just started. I hummed along with the music from Barry Manilow's song, '*When will our eyes meet? When can I touch you? When will this strong yearning end? When will I hold you again?*'

The music was as comforting as when I was a child and would nestle at my mother's feet with my back pressed against the vibrating piano.

I needed both of my hands to push the foot pedal to the floor.

'Don't touch,' my mother would barely whisper. She wouldn't open her eyes.

'I'm helping you,' I would say, sitting cross-legged on the carpet by her feet.

She wouldn't respond, so I'd watch her arms move back and forth across the piano keys. Left and right. Right and left. They floated when the music was soft. They were stiff and firm when she played the keys loudly. I rested my hand on top of her right foot, the one closest to me, so my hand could ride up and down as she pressed the foot pedals, and I could be nearer to her.

'Stop,' she'd say. Sometimes she didn't speak softly.

I would push the palms of my hands against the carpet and

scoot back to lean against the piano's blond wood etched with dark grain lines, and I'd feel as well as hear the sounds. White felt-tipped arms rose and fell inside the piano. I'd seen the arms move when my mother raised the lid to retrieve a hairbrush or book or pencil that my brothers or I had dropped inside. With the top raised, she would move her fingers across the keyboard sounding one key at a time until she heard the one or ones whose sounds were muted or distorted by something as big as a magazine or as small as a Popsicle stick. Then she'd reach into the workings of the piano to retrieve the offending object.

Loving her music was the same as loving her, I would discover. I loved the trills, with harmonies played mostly on black keys, the only ones that worked on the old piano in a neighbor's garage where my mother taught herself to play by ear when she was a child. She was the music: the variations of melodies that were flights far from the original or deliciously similar. She was the whole orchestra; she played all the parts. 'Here are the violins. Now the horns,' she'd announce. She interpreted melodies by adding ornamentation, altering tones, a whole or half note apart or scaling through a series of consecutive tones all to explain or explore the emotions, the intricacies of expression. Sometimes my mother would play songs I knew well and mis-play parts. I'd whip my head around to look at her and she'd grin and say, 'Just wondered if you were listening.' I knew her moods through her music. They ranged from Cole Porter's *Begin the Beguine* to the song that reminded her of her mother's funeral, Claude Debussy's *Clare de Lune*. For a time, I thought that when people played the piano, they could no longer hear the phone or the doorbell or see their children. For a time, I thought that everyone's mother played so many renditions of *Happy Birthday* that they had to be asked to stop before the ice cream melted. In time, I would learn that my mother's far-away look had a name: passion.

Tom came into my hospital room carrying two large Styrofoam cups in his hands. Dangling from his teeth was a small brown paper bag.

'Food. Oh, my gosh. Thanks. What did you find to eat?'

'Mumm hun,' he mumbled, the bag still dangling from his clenched teeth. 'Corned beef sandwiches with sauerkraut,' he said when he'd put the Styrofoam cups full of coffee on the bedside table and had taken the bag from his teeth.

'At 5.30 in the morning?'

'The cafeteria won't be open till 6.00. I found these in a machine in the nurses' lounge downstairs,' he said, pulling containers of cream from his pants pocket. 'Here, two for you, one for me. Oh, I almost forgot. I brought a pint of milk for the nursing mother,' he said, digging into his other pants pocket.

I bit the wrapper with my teeth to tear the cellophane. 'I didn't know a sandwich from a machine could taste this good.'

'Nothing like hard labor to build an appetite.'

'We can't even call anyone. It's too early,' I mumbled between bites of corned beef and thick rye bread.

'There won't be any Boy Scouts at our house. No father/son camping trips,' the former scoutmaster said.

'Give me a chance and I'll have the three boys next. But please, next time get somebody to do something more than tell me to push. I needed some painkillers. That wasn't right. I hurt too much.'

'What could I do?'

'Back me up. Insist on some medicine.'

'You know, three girls are enough to educate and to care for.'

'I know. But I'll miss it all when it's over. The nuzzling, suckling, baby smiles, cooing to call me before she knows words, the giggles when you touch ticklish spots. "Tickling ribs" my mother calls them.'

'Night feedings. Days when you don't get anything else done but baby. No nice dinner for the husband.'

'It won't be long and we can start calling people. Who do we know who gets up early? Carol. She never sleeps more than five hours a night. She's probably awake. If not, she wouldn't be upset if I woke her. Or she wouldn't let me know that she was upset.'

'Let's at least wait until 6.00 a.m.'

From 6.00 until nearly 8.00, we called Molly and Emily, our parents, Carl and Pete, Tom's parents, his brothers, John and Pete, sister, Barb, and friends whom we knew well enough to wake on a Sunday morning.

'I thought you said we might have a boy this time,' Molly said.

'When can you come home with her, Mom?' Emily asked.

'As soon as the doctor checks her honey. About 10.00 a.m. . . . Daddy will come to Grammie's house and get you and Molly. Then we can all ride home together. Are you having fun? You're eating pancakes shaped like Mickey Mouse with big ears? Emily, that's great. I love you. Yes, I know it's a long wait until ten o'clock. Aren't there any cartoons on TV? Oh, you're right.

It is Sunday, isn't it? Maybe you can help Grammie wash dishes. Oh, you think you may be able to find something else to do until 10.00? Okay, good girl.'

My mother and I talked about Sarah's birth date being May 3 and what a tribute it was to the memory of my brother Joe, who was born on that date also. While he lived, my brother Joe was one of my favorites because as a young boy, he was soft and kind and entertaining. Even before he could say words, he would stand on the coffee table and babble and wave his arms and hold our attention with his smiles and laughter and flirtatious eyes. My mother called him 'The Politician'. Later when he did say a few words, he'd announce the beginning of a speech, 'Wadies and gemewen.'

Joe baited us with his eyes and a grin that promised fun and mischief. His body in motion was also eye-catching. He was a natural sportsman like our father. He whistled happy tunes. Joe was a junior at the University of California at Davis when Mom got a call from a campus police officer. Joe's van was found with one end of plastic tubing taped to the van's tailpipe. The other end was pushed into the driver's side window; the window was open just enough to let the hose in. Joe was inside, dead. I told Mom that his suffering was over. She cried saying that she didn't know he was suffering. True. None of knew he was sad, or hurting, or suicidal. Sarah was born five years later.

It was 4.00 a.m. in California, so my mother offered to call my brothers Frank and Mike later in the morning. At 8.00 a.m. Tom left to get Molly and Emily and bring them back to the hospital to see their sister and bring us home. Tom gave me a quick business-like kiss. That's when I saw his shoulders droop the way they do when he's tired. He hadn't left my side all night. He must have used the bathroom or gotten a drink of water sometime during the night, but I didn't remember a moment without him. And I didn't remember him complaining of being tired, or of his back hurting as it does when he sits too long.

I watched the parking lot and the highway in front of the hospital that skirted the coast of North Carolina. I searched for our Volvo among the cars that left the hospital parking lot. Probably 30 cars left the lot. I didn't see Tom or our car. I wanted to.

Ocean freighters were docked for loading just across the street from the hospital. The sunrise behind them outlined their length from bow to stern. It was a different way to watch the ocean.

Mostly my view was of a beach full of swimmers, sunbathers, and seagulls. But here, there was no beach, and a full view of the water was blocked by storage containers marked Texaco and Exxon and piles of cartons labeled Chiquita. Although I couldn't read the writing, the trademark picture of the banana was large enough to see from my window. Cranes lifted massive bundles that began to sway as they were maneuvered from the dock to the cargo ships. Seamen delivered cargo and loaded ships for another trip at sea. They'll have their adventure; I'll have mine with a new baby.

'*When will our eyes meet? When can I touch you? When will I hold you again?*' Sleep would not come, so I closed my eyes and listened to the music.

Breakfast of eggs, bacon, toast, orange juice, and coffee arrived. It was hot but the portions were small. I could have eaten it again. I didn't fill out the lunch menu because I would be eating lunch at home.

At 9.30 a.m., I walked into the hall. A nurse carried a new baby to its mother in a room past mine. After the nursery, my room was the first patient's room.

'Has the neonatologist come to the hospital yet this morning?' I called after the nurse.

'Yes, he has.'

Good, I thought, I got back into bed and fluffed up a couple of pillows: one to lean against and one to prop under my arm to support Sarah while she nursed.

I had only met the neonatologist once. I was about seven months pregnant when my obstetrician asked me who would be caring for the new baby. I didn't know any doctors in the city where our third child would be born. I'd only come to the city to have the baby so I could use the obstetrician who was in favor of prepared childbirth. The pediatrician we regularly used lived in the same town we did and was on staff at the hospital there, so he couldn't look after our third child after she was born.

'Who do you use?' I asked the father of four whose fifth baby was due a week after mine. It didn't seem too personal a question, so I was surprised when he didn't answer. 'Who would you recommend?' I tried again wondering why he was reluctant to respond.

'We have no pediatricians in town, but we are fortunate to have a neonatologist, a specialist in newborn care, here at our small hospital. His office is in the next building,' he motioned, pointing out the window to another set of office buildings. 'Why don't you try to see him today before you go home?'

Although the recommendation was a bit guarded, I went to the neonatologist's office that day. He was too busy to see me then but could see me a month later.

'Why are you here? I see infants and children, not mothers,' the neonatologist said, staring at the eighth-month bulge under my maternity dress. He was a small man, in his mid-40s probably, and rather nondescript. I stood in the doorway to his office while he sat at his desk. Maybe it was the sun's glare from the window behind him, but from where I stood, his hair appeared to be so close to the color of his skin that it was difficult to tell where his forehead ended and his hair began.

My gut-reaction was to find another doctor. But it had taken a month to get an appointment to meet him, and the baby was due in just over three weeks. So I decided to put his personality aside and trust his expertise, as all I needed was someone to examine the baby then we'd both be home hours after delivery.

The second time I saw the neonatologist, he walked into my room, came right up to my bed and said, 'Your baby has a slight breathing problem. Premature. She'll outgrow it.'

'When can I see her?'

'At the next feeding at noon,' he said, turning to leave.

'But, doctor, wait,' I called after him. He held onto the doorframe as if to hold himself back. 'My baby's not premature. I know my dates. I tried for two and a half years to get pregnant. I know my dates.'

'She's premature.'

And he was gone from the doorway. I walked to the nursery across the hall to see Sarah. A wide shade was pulled down almost to the bottom edge of the nursery window. By bending down and looking up, I could see Sarah. She was sleeping. I watched her chest rise and fall quickly, but not too quickly. She looked peaceful. It must have been quite warm in the room, as she didn't have a shirt on. A 6 lb baby would be skinny, I thought, but Sarah wasn't. She was round and pink. Her legs, feet, arms, and hands were perfectly formed, as were her tiny features: tipped nose, dark eyelashes. Her dark reddish hair, the color of antique mahogany, was stunning. My empty arms ached to hold her. A nurse inside the nursery motioned me away as she pulled on the end of the shade.

'I'm the mother,' I said, pointing to Sarah. 'May I hold her?'

'No, no. She's to stay in the nursery.'

'I'll come in and hold her in there,' I told her as I walked toward the door. I saw an extra rocking chair that I could use.

'I can't let you in here. And I must pull the shade. It's not viewing time.'

I could bring a chair from my room, I thought, and place it under the window. From that angle I could look at Sarah through the thin space between the end of the shade and the bottom of the window, and I wouldn't have to bend over. But the nurse pulled the shade all the way down. And I couldn't see Sarah at all.

There was no harmony to the music anymore, just piano keys plaintively tapping out the discordant notes one-by-one. In my hospital room, I sat on the edge of the bed and pushed buttons on the remote control. Station after station showed the Sunday preachers, some robed, some in suits. Some stood in front of choirs adorned with satiny gold and blue graduation-style gowns. The preachers waved their arms theatrically or held up their hands in earnest as they chanted Bible verses and admonished viewers to renounce Satan and mail their checks to this station. TV religion was not something I watched. I hadn't even been to church in years. I clicked off the remote.

I called Tom. 'Don't come to get me yet. Sarah has a minor breathing problem. I'll get her at noon.'

Somehow noon arrived, not aided by my clock watching or my pacing. A nurse carried a hungry baby to its mother. The baby cried. It was not Sarah's cry. Who was hungrier, I wondered, mothers or babies? From my bulging breasts to my pounding heart, my body longed for Sarah. My stomach was as nervous as if I were waiting for my first date. The neonatologist leaned into my room to say that Sarah would be staying in the nursery, that I still couldn't hold her or feed her. 'She's fine – just this breathing problem particular to preemies. You can have her for the next feeding at three.' He turned and headed down the hall.

'But she's not premature,' I said, too loudly. I didn't mean to yell. The nicer I am, the quicker I can hold Sarah again. But the damage was done. The doctor took a few steps backward, turned to face me, and frowned.

'I'll be out of town this afternoon. I'm flying my plane.'

My hospital bed was in an upright position, so I could sit up and nurse. The pillows for propping up my elbows while I cradled Sarah were on the bed. Sarah had missed three feedings. My breasts ached. I wrapped my arms around them and cried.

6. Eighteen hours

The door to my hospital room opened with a bang as it slammed into the doorstop. A man in jeans and a red and black flannel shirt was at the foot of my bed.

'I'm Dr Smith. I'm the doctor on call for your neonatologist. You have a sick daughter.'

'You mean the minor breathing problem?'

'I suspect pneumonia. I need your permission to take chest X-rays.'

'Sure,' I heard myself say.

He left the room as quickly as he entered, saying, 'Don't panic. I'll tell you when to panic.'

Minutes later he was back. Sarah had pneumonia. Could he do a spinal tap? I nodded.

'How is she?' I asked.

'She is on the critical list. But babies can get sick very quickly and recover just as quickly. It's not time to panic yet.'

I called Tom and my mother. 'She's going to be all right. She's on the critical list. But Dr Smith thinks she'll recover quickly.'

Dr Smith was in my room again. 'Sarah has sepsis, a blood infection. She's on antibiotics and a ventilator. Don't panic yet. I'll tell you when to panic.'

I stared into his eyes to learn what he was thinking. I wanted to know what he knew about babies who had pneumonia and sepsis. And what he thought about Sarah. But all I saw in his eyes was compassion, and it scared me.

'Let me hold her, please.'

'No.'

'Let me look at her, please.'

'No.'

Dr Smith's beeper went off, and he left the room in his now characteristic run.

My phone rang. 'This is Dr Smith. I need your permission to do an electrocardiogram.'

STAT to the nursery. Beep-beep-beep, the hospital intercom sounded.

Dr Smith was in the doorway of my room. Sarah had had a heart attack. But she was stable. It was three o'clock, time for another feeding, when Dr Smith ran from my room. This time he didn't tell me not to panic.

My brother Little Joe was born and died of a weak heart, and another brother Pete was born with heart problems and for the first weeks of his life, he wasn't expected to live. The words *heart attack* catapulted my mind to a possibility I dared not imagine. I lay in limbo. If my fingers gripped the satiny bindings of the blanket or my arms crushed a pillow full of feathers to my chest or my legs paced my body around the room like a wounded animal, I don't know. I have no memory of the afternoon turning to evening.

It was dark outside when the neonatologist poked his head into my room. 'Call your husband. Tell him to come here,' he said.

I don't remember if I called Tom. Shock is so consuming that it leaves little room for memory.

How could I have a sick child? I took prenatal vitamins, saw the obstetrician monthly and at the end, weekly. I didn't eat junk food. All the signs were good: blood tests, urine tests, blood pressure, growth rates. I even stopped working two weeks ago so that I could take more naps.

In some ways this pregnancy had been better than the others because this obstetrician had no problem with my gaining 40 lbs. With the others, doctors had thought that 40 lbs was too much to gain, so they asked me how many extra pounds would I like to carry around in memory of this pregnancy? Or did I know that any weight I gained over 18 lbs would make a bigger baby and cause delivery to be more difficult? This obstetrician mentioned at one office visit that I had gained 7 lbs that month. 'Don't you think that's a lot?' he asked. When I told him that it was all vegetables, fruit, and fish and that I'd never had any trouble getting back to my normal 125 lbs, he just smiled. That was our last discussion about weight gain.

I was more tired during that third pregnancy. And nausea lasted longer. But I also worked full time and cared for two young children. Perhaps being tired and experiencing bouts of nausea were to be expected. No, those weren't signs of a troubled pregnancy.

'I've got some good news and some bad news for you,' the neonatologist was saying as he stood in the center of my room for one of his give-the-message-and-leave visits. 'Before that, let me tell you, you have a sick baby. Now the good news: we have some excellent hospitals to care for sick babies. The bad news is that there is no room in any of those hospitals, so we're taking your baby to the hospital in Wilmington. It's 70 miles from here. They are better equipped there than we are to care for your baby.'

Two nurses came in, one older, one younger. 'Come with us,' the older one said. 'You can see your baby now.' I couldn't see her when I wanted to. I had begged for 15 hours to hold her, feed her, look at her. Now the nurses were telling me to look at her. The shift scared me.

'What does she look like?'

'There's a tube going into her navel and wires taped to her chest and tubes in her nose, needles in her feet, and tubes running from them,' a nurse said.

'She's in pain, isn't she?' I asked. 'And no one is holding her.'

'Oh, I held her this afternoon, and I fed her her bottle,' the younger nurse said brightly.

Why couldn't I have held her, fed her? I wasn't allowed even to look at her. No one realized she was sick until she was very sick. If I had been able to see her, I would have known something was wrong. I could have done something. I could have gotten another doctor. I told the neonatologist that she wasn't premature. He never listened to me. He thought he knew what was wrong with Sarah without listening to me.

I wondered what my face looked like because the nurses were staring at me with an expression I was to see often in the next few years. It's the same look I got when I told people that my baby brother, Little Joe, had died and later another brother, Robert, who never came home from the hospital, and after my dad's death, and after another brother, Joe, died. It's the same look you see on the faces of people on the side of the road or in the median of a freeway as they stare into their wrecked cars. You wonder what they are seeing. Then you drive by and see the blood-red sheet covering the human shape or you see an arm dangling or head slumped across the steering wheel, and you don't wonder anymore.

'They are going to put her in the ambulance in a few minutes. Come and see her,' the older nurse said.

Years later as I think about those two nurses urging me to see Sarah, I know that was the moment my limbo ended. I entered the leading edge of an emotional maelstrom that my mother knew times three, when she began to realize that her children were dead or dying. I'd spent a lifetime trying to ensure that I would never go there. Yet I was helpless to stop what was happening. I could do nothing for Sarah. I could only save myself from seeing her once-relaxed little face lined with evidence of pain, her body assaulted with tubes and needles and bruised from repeated needle sticks, her chest reddened by the machine that both shocked her heart into restarting and perhaps cracked some ribs as well, and her chest heaving with pneumonia's labored breathing. I shook my head. The nurses left my room.

Another nurse came in saying, 'Wilmington always calls when our babies arrive. We'll let you know as soon as they call us.'

The neonatologist stood in my room. He looked at me with the same expression on his face that the nurses had. Had I turned into a freak? 'Let me know when you hear something,' I said. 'I don't want to be the last to know what's going on.'

I took off my nightgown and put on the maternity dress I'd brought to wear home. I couldn't think about Sarah being sick; I concentrated on the design of the dress that my friend Lindy had loaned me. The dress fell in folds from my shoulders. It had a rounded collar, a short buttoned placket opening at the neck, and short puffed sleeves that ended in narrow fitted cuffs. But the beauty of the dress was in the folds of fabric that cascaded out and down to soften the abrupt bulge of pregnancy and now to let me leave the hospital with dignity even though I had 17 lbs to lose. I packed my overnight bag. There was no reason to stay in the hospital. Sarah wasn't here. As I put my address book, the last of my things, in my bag, my obstetrician came into my room.

'Where do you think you're going?' he asked. 'We're still trying to find out what made your baby sick.'

'I'm going home,' I told him. Yet I hadn't called anyone for a ride. I didn't have a car at the hospital. It was too far to walk. How disorienting shock is.

'You need to stay here,' the doctor said. 'You are going to be treated too. We don't want you to get whatever your baby has.'

I changed back into my nightgown to wait for news that Sarah had arrived safely and that doctors had begun treatment to help her fight the illness, whatever it was.

I called Tom to tell him the doctor would be treating me so that I wouldn't get whatever it was that was making Sarah sick. I wanted him with me, but I don't know if I asked him to come. Tom asked me to keep him informed, so I knew he wasn't coming. Maybe he told me that it was so late that visiting hours would be over by the time he could get to the hospital. He wouldn't have questioned the hospital's policy on visiting hours.

After Molly and Emily were born, Tom made obligatory visits

to the hospital to see me in the evenings after work. He wouldn't sit but would pace uncomfortably until I'd ask him if he wanted to leave. He would. He's not much for small talk or handholding, and in the early years of women's lib, it wasn't masculine to dote, and certainly not publicly. If Tom had come to the hospital when Sarah was sick, it would have been his idea and not an obligation. If I had asked him to come, I might have thought about his being uncomfortable. I was too needy to care for someone else. Years later, as I recalled those hours in the hospital, those hours that would cast shadows and lights on all the years and hopes and ambitions and sorrows that followed, I wondered if I asked him to come, and he told me that he was putting the girls to bed. Shock has a poor memory.

I used to be jealous of friends whose husbands sat with them in their hospital rooms for hours after work, watching television or just sitting in the room reading or chatting about what had come in the mail or what the kids had done that day or how many ounces of formula the newborn had consumed, how many diapers she'd wet or pooped. Then I'd hear stories of the same men having affairs, and I decided I'd rather have my husband than ones who'd visit their wives in the hospital and visit their girlfriends as well. It hurt, though, as appearances were all too important in those early years of marriage. When a fellow mid-level manager at Tom's company would buy a new family car, the rest of us would get new car-itis. We wanted to look equally prosperous, although we were all making about the same salaries. How well our children were dressed or how quickly they learned to read reflected, we thought, upon the strengths of our parenting abilities. I would fantasize in those beginning years of our marriage – when the name-brand clothes our children wore had been purchased at yard sales – that I was beyond looks, that yard-sale clothes made it possible for me to stay home with them until they went to preschool, that our children would make us proud, that even though Tom didn't take me out to romantic dinners, he realized how important staying home with the children was to me. He was providing me with something greater than the appearance of romance, more than a show for other couples. I'd fantasize while I looked at those husbands who brought boxes of candy to their wives in confinement following childbirth that our marriage would grow stronger, that we had something better than a romantic look.

Tom didn't know that the terror I was experiencing in the hospital when Sarah was ill was exponentially increased by my being alone, and no one from the hospital called to tell him to come or to inform him that the baby's health was rapidly deteriorating. I was not relating information correctly or adequately and neither of us was prepared for a sick child. Had Tom known how sick Sarah was or if he'd had experience with death and the close-but-no-comparison – near death – he would have been with me.

The phone at the nurses' station had rung every few minutes all day. When the door to my room was opened, I could hear the phone ring and hear the nurses talking. Often the voices were muffled and the words were difficult to understand because of the noises of hospital carts being pushed or the elevator doors opening and shutting with a metal clang. But I could hear the phone ringing, and I could hear the nurses answer the phone. Even if I couldn't distinguish the words, the lilt in their voices would tell me when the news was good.

I opened the door to the hall, turned off the light, lay on top of the blanket, and waited for the phone to ring. I would know that Sarah was at the hospital in Wilmington even before the nurse came to tell me. The phone didn't ring. I waited until it was dark outside, and I saw the neonatologist standing in the doorway to my room.

The light from behind him made his body a faceless silhouette. He had said he would tell me when he knew anything. And there he was. All the other times he had come to talk about Sarah, he had come into the room or at least stuck his head into the room. Now he stood in the doorway. I sat up quickly, awakened by his presence from fitful, fearful dozing. I stared at his shape and I waited. But there was nothing. No throat clearing. Not a gasp. Not even a sigh. I waited for a lifetime, afraid of what he might say.

'She's dead,' I said finally.

'Yes,' he said.

'Why?'

'You didn't come to the hospital soon enough.'

I didn't have any skin on. I could tell without looking. It hurt to breathe. As I inhaled, my lungs expanded, exposing more of my insides to the air. The air stung. Muscle fibers thin as hair glistened. They dried and died as they were exposed to air. I took shallow breaths and the pain lessened. The doctor's silhouette remained in the doorway, intrusive as an onlooker at the scene of a tragedy.

'Close the door on your way out,' I told him.

I lay in the hospital bed and felt my cells dying from the outside in, layer by layer by layer. Deeper and deeper. The pain ebbed and flowed from intolerable to excruciating. My body was dying. I waited for the nerve cells to stop transmitting messages of pain. I lay motionless, barely breathing, waiting for death to stop the pain.

'Here's a pill,' a nurse said as she handed me a plastic cup.

I shook my head and turned my back to her.

'It's a tranquilizer. You must take it.'

'No.' I do not have to take a pill. A pill would make me sleep. To sleep a drugged sleep and wake up to this again would be a nightmare. I will not stop the process only to start it again when the tranquilizer wears off. No, I will lie here and feel my cells dying.

She left. Another nurse came into my room. She brought the plastic cup with the pill in it and a box of Kleenex. She put the box of Kleenex on my bed and sat down next to it.

'You can cry now,' she said.

'I don't feel like crying,' I told her.

'Then take the pill.'

'No.'

She left.

The room was dark. I lay in bed and tried to think of reasons to live. Without Sarah, I could think of none. Mentally, I said goodbye to my family: my uncles and aunts and cousins, my brothers, my mother, my daughters. I tried to say goodbye to Tom but I couldn't. I couldn't focus on what it was that I couldn't let go. I just couldn't say goodbye to him yet. I imagined his fingers brushing away my tears, and his arms holding me close to him, the tenderness and the firmness together coaxing my body to live. My mind swirled, wanting to give in to death and imagining the warmth and weight of Tom's arms.

'Call your husband. Tell him to come here,' someone was saying.

My fingers dialed the numbers.

'We can have another baby,' Tom was saying. 'Keep a stiff upper lip . . . When can you come home? . . . What do I tell the girls when they wake up?'

I couldn't focus on his questions enough to answer them. I don't remember responding.

'When is he coming?' a nurse asked when I put the receiver down.

'I don't know. Our daughters are asleep.'

'Then call your mother. Tell her to come.'

The phone woke my mother. I heard her fumbling for her glasses and the light switch on the tall tiffany lamp by her bed.

'The baby's dead. Would you come and pick me up? I want to go home . . . Yes, please come now.'

After I put the receiver down, the nurse picked up the box of Kleenex and the cup with the pill and left.

Another nurse came into the room. 'You need to do something with the body. What are your plans?'

I opened my mouth to speak but nothing happened. I hadn't thought of my baby being a body.

'We can't keep it in the morgue past tomorrow morning,' she said, tossing the words over her shoulder as she turned and walked out of the room.

I tried not to breathe. It hurt to breathe.

The nurse-midwife came right up to the side of my bed, pressing her thigh against the mattress. She leaned down, put her face close to mine and said in a loud whisper, 'You were only thinking of yourself.' Then she turned abruptly and left the room.

Whatever could she mean? Mean, meanness. She means meanness. Why?

My obstetrician and a nurse came.

'She's never lost a baby before,' he said of his nurse-midwife. I wondered what that had to do with anything. I wondered if I was supposed to feel something for her. I've never lost a baby either. It wasn't her baby. It was mine. Moments later, giving voice to empathy, he asked, 'How are you?'

'I have grieved before,' I said, 'my father and three brothers.' Their deaths, I imagined, had prepared me for what was ahead. In reality, grieving for them was far shorter and less intense than what I would experience in the months and years ahead. Paradoxically, it would be another decade before the medical community would begin to realize that the death of an infant, or stillbirth or miscarriage, was a loss worthy of grief. The medical prescription, the salve, the comfort for a baby's death then was: dismiss it, move on. Even kind hearted physicians would tell their patients and their own daughters to stop crying, to get on with life, to have another baby, and to take care of the loved ones they had. Community members, neighbors, friends by extrapolation – taking cues from learned physicians – believed that the death of a baby was a blip in the road of life; potholes happen, don't look back, keep driving. So mothers, fathers, siblings, grandparents experienced emotions that were not validated. At the times when emotional support was crucial to reconnecting with life and becoming whole and healthy again, friends and family – acting on the best medical knowledge at the time – were for the most part absent, because they didn't think these deaths were anything to cry about.

My obstetrician and his nurse were on either side of my hospital bed ready to escort me to an examining room. 'We need to grow some cultures,' the doctor said. 'We're trying to find out why your baby got sick.'

It doesn't matter now. It mattered when she was alive.

'Your baby may have picked up a bacteria or virus from you before she was born. You could develop the same disease. We need to start cultures growing to decide how to treat you.'

I didn't care if I got sick or died. The doctor was beside me. The nurse was on my other side. My legs were walking me out of the room and into another room, one with an examining table. My heels were in the metal stirrups.

'This will hurt,' he said. 'I don't like to do this so soon after delivery.'

I didn't feel anything. Maybe my definition of pain had changed. Maybe I couldn't feel anymore. I saw long, cotton-tipped sticks go from the doctor's hand to the nurse's.

When he finished, he lifted my legs out of the stirrups gently. Never before had a doctor lifted my legs out of the stirrups. It was a small thing, but I felt like crying when he took his hands off my legs. It was the first touch, the first time I had felt someone else's skin since the baby died.

The urge to cry vanished and in its place was a feeling of violation. I was violated by vaginal exams throughout three pregnancies, four miscarriages, and years of infertility. I was violated, too, by the neonatologist, by nurses, by disease, by death. Nothing I had submitted to or worked for or prayed for the past three and a half years had given me the baby I wanted. I was dying of violation, but that touch was harder to bear because it connected me with a person – it connected me with living. I didn't cry, but it had been easier to keep my emotions from welling up before that touch.

Walking out of the examining room, the nurse and the doctor were on either side of me. The floor swelled and the walls swayed from a night of labor rather than sleep and 18 hours of longing and fear. In bed, fatigue and weakness came in a rush. I heard the doctor's voice as I drifted in and out of a fog and into a nightmare.

Your baby died of a heart attack . . . before she was admitted . . . Wilmington is a teaching hospital . . . wise to have an autopsy . . . it could have been done for free had your baby been admitted. We don't know what caused your baby's death . . . could have been a genetic problem – heart maybe. Knowing what caused her death may affect your decision to have more children.

Not have more children? We want another child.

We don't know what caused your baby's death. The neonatologist said it was my fault she died. The nurse-midwife had said that I was only thinking of myself as if I had something to do with her death. This doctor is saying he doesn't know why she died. An autopsy could prove that I did not cause her death. Two of my brothers had congenital heart problems. Sarah could have had heart trouble. We don't know why she died. We don't know. Don't know yet. Wait for contractions. If it's a girl, Sarah. If it's a boy, Josh. Rest. Need to be rested. Long night ahead. I'm so tired. Can't go into labor this tired.

A scream – a long, low, monotonic sound like a loud moan ripped through the quiet. It was the sound of terror. The scream grew louder. I was afraid of what I would know when I found where the scream was coming from. I was afraid of discovering horror. I was afraid of what I would learn about pain if I were to find out who was screaming and why. I opened my eyes. It was dark outside. My cheeks were wet. I didn't know why. I wiped. The wet was from my tears.

Oh, my God. Sarah. Not my Sarah. Not my baby. Please, God.

PART 2

7. Night and day

The girls were asleep when I told Tom that Sarah died. He hung the phone's receiver on the kitchen wall but didn't release his hand immediately. The words *dead* and *baby* set off internal alarms and explosions. His head hurt. His stomach lurched. His body rose off the kitchen stool, and his hands clutched his head as if to stop the throbbing. He paced in wide circular motions toward the refrigerator, toward the stove, toward the window overlooking the backyard now black as the night sky. His arms found a wall and his fists pounded. He stopped only after realizing that his hands ached. He alternately opened and closed his fists to shake out the ache and see if his fingers still worked. He swung open a cabinet door and reached for a bottle of scotch; from another cabinet he pulled a glass off a shelf. He poured clear brown liquid in a glass, added ice and water, took a swallow, and felt the burn. It was only then, minutes after the phone call, that he remembered the girls. He looked at his watch. In a few hours, they would wake. They would be expecting to go to the hospital to pick up their mommy and new baby sister. A wail he hardly recognized as his own pierced the quiet. His arms cradled his head, and his shoulders shook as he sobbed.

Sometime before midnight, he called my mother.

'Miz,' he said, his voice unnaturally hoarse and deeper than normal. He breathed by inhaling in gulps.

'Tom, how are you?' She asked what she already knew. She'd answered the phone in the kitchen where she was heating water to make instant coffee before driving to the hospital with Pete and Carl.

'I don't know. Okay.'

'Are the girls asleep?'

'Yes.'

'Good,' she said, pouring bubbling hot water into a coffee cup.

'The girls are going to wake up and I . . .' He gulped for air.

My mother's voice was steady, confident, strong, as she is. She is best in times of crisis. It's years later that she cries, becomes depressed, and doesn't know why. She was 16 when her mother died; her father didn't or couldn't provide a safe environment for her to grieve. So she delays her own grief while sustaining family and friends through their toughest times.

'Just tell them that Sarah got sick and died. Then answer their questions. Expect any reaction. If they cry, hold them. If they don't seem to comprehend the information, just go with it. Children can't take it all in – what dead means. They have no basis for understanding the concept.'

'But they are so excited. I mean, they went to bed so happy. I told them that Sarah got sick, but none of us thought that this would happen. We all thought T and Sarah would be home in the morning.'

I didn't dare sleep that night. Couldn't sleep. I walked the halls. Starting at my bed, I walked by the sink and out the door into the hall. To the right was the nurses' station, to the left were hospital rooms. One room had a mother in it whose baby was alive. I went to the right. I wished the hall were longer. As short as it was, I must have walked in front of the nurses' station a hundred times before my mother and Carl and Pete arrived.

My mother's arms were around me. My brother Carl was hugging me. My brother Pete held both of my hands in his own. Their skin covered my dying, skinless body until the stinging stopped and I could breathe again. Please, I thought, don't ever let go.

They stayed with me until I was discharged later the next afternoon. Maybe the hospital's strict visiting hours didn't apply if someone died. Nurses wheeled a rollaway bed into my room for my mother. Carl stretched out on the extra bed. Pete pushed two peacock-blue vinyl chairs together so that sitting up he could stretch his legs out and sleep, sort of. We each had a pillow since I had brought extra ones for nursing. Sometimes I thought I had slept, but I would open my eyes to look at my mother or my brothers. One of them would feel me looking at them and wake up and say, 'Hi, sis,' or, 'Oh, T.'

That's all that was said. Sometimes we didn't say anything; we just waved at each other from across the room. Their voices and little waves made by raising fingers off the pillow or mattress and moving them in a semi-circle until they came down to rest again on the pillow or mattress kept me alive that night. Soon it was morning, and we didn't have to pretend to be sleeping. That's how my obstetrician found us.

'I'm ordering you an antibiotic. Your baby died of a strep infection. Group Beta streptococcus.'

'What is that?' I asked.

'A bacteria that caused an infection.'

'Then she picked it up from the hospital?'

'No, she picked it up from you. That's why you must be treated. So you don't get sick too.'

Tom slept a little but woke before the alarm. He toasted bread for Emily, spread butter on it, and sprinkled cinnamon and sugar. For Molly he filled a cereal bowl with Cheerios. Then he poured two glasses of orange juice.

Tom was the better parent to tell the girls. He was calm. He didn't cry. A parent's tears might have frightened them. He was stoic – the only way he knows – like his Bostonian mother. I asked him once, after his beloved grandfather died, why he didn't appear to feel the sadness. 'What good would it do? It won't change the outcome.' Stoic, I'm not; I'm more like my Irish than my German ancestors – my highs and lows are passionate, palpable, thin-skinned.

Months and years later I would envision the girls hearing of Sarah's death: the little faces showing a range of emotions, then their bodies acting them out, then the withdrawal alternating with the lashing out at life when it's most brutal. All the anticipation of this baby's long-awaited birth, shattered.

'Sarah won't be coming home,' Tom told Molly when she woke up. Molly had many questions. How did she get sick? Why couldn't doctors make her well? When could she see Sarah? When is Mommy coming home? Why did she get sick? Then she cried and climbed into his lap. After a hug, she went into her bedroom and kicked her stuffed animals. Tom followed her, telling her he thought she should go to school so she would have something to do.

Emily listened while Molly asked questions and Tom answered them. Then she told her daddy she was going to go back to sleep. After a few minutes, she came out of her bedroom and asked if she could watch TV. She watched cartoons, but she was agitated. She gathered her Acey, her security blanket, around her face, fingered a corner, sucked her thumb, then smoothed Acey until it covered her curled-up legs, then gathered it again and clutched it. She repeated the movements over and over.

Had I been making the decision instead of Tom, I probably would have kept Molly home from school that day, for what I'm not sure: to protect her maybe, or to shield myself from having to see my friends and coworkers as I dropped her off or picked her up. Sitting at home, hearing the phone ring, answering the door as neighbors came with gifts of food and florists dropped off flowers and potted plants would not have been action enough for Molly. So Tom probably made the right decision. Life for Molly is not a spectator sport. Nor is it something to ponder. It is for diving into. For the first five years of her life I was Molly's entertainment committee. 'I'm bored,' she'd say as she'd finish putting a puzzle together or finish cutting out shapes and gluing them to a piece of cardboard. After she learned to read, she could entertain herself for longer periods of time. Sending her to school that day was probably for the best.

At the elementary school on that Monday morning, Tom kept the Volvo's engine running as he reached behind him to flip the back door's lock open. Molly gripped the handle of her lunch box in one hand and the strap of her backpack in the other hand. 'Bye, hon,' he said.

'Are you picking me up?' she asked.

'Yes, I think so,' he told her.

So, Molly was the one who told the teachers, my coworkers, about Sarah. Their hands covering their open mouths, the jaws that fell open of their own volition without the owner's knowledge or forethought. The physical reactions scared her. The teachers would have inhaled air with those open mouths as they tried to take in the unnatural, the unexpected, the too-close-to-home news. Their voices would have been unnaturally high, 'Are you serious?' Or, 'What happened?' There she would have been at seven years old watching her teachers, my friends, stunned, so soon after they had surprised me with the baby shower. After taking in the news, they slipped easily into teacher-mode, and hugged her until she was emotionally her normal, confident self.

That demeanor would last until a look, a word, a thought of the death would pierce her world again and again. She grieved as a child grieves, taking in the reality in pieces or pierces throughout childhood until she could finally process the death as an adult.

Emily stayed home from playschool. Unlike Molly, she would have needed to be in her most familiar, secure place. She sat on the sofa in the living room clutching her Acey. The television stayed on, the volume low. She looked at the picture but didn't process the cartoons; she was processing something more important: things weren't going as planned.

Early in the afternoon on that Monday, I was released from the hospital and into a world different from the one I'd left three days before. Even the air was different; everything was hazy as if fog were attempting to fill a void. The haze muted colors to grays, whites, and blacks. It muffled voices making them difficult to understand. Cloud-like and billowing, it seeped easily into my skinless body. I was becoming lighter as I became more fog than me. The daylight made my eyes burn and water.

There was less light in the back seat of my mother's yellow VW, so I got in back. Carl drove. Pete sat next to him. My mother sat in back with me. She put her hand over my knee and pressed with her fingers. Want to know how a crow lights? She'd ask us when we were young and giggly. Sure, we'd bite, feigning ignorance. Then those fingers would reach across the couch or to the chair where one of us was sitting and grip a knee, and she'd increase the pressure until we squealed and begged her to stop – all the while hoping she wouldn't. Mimicking her physician-grandmother's physical exams, she'd have us sit down and cross our legs and use her flat hand as a doctor's rubber hammer, palm up/fingers out straight and pressed together, to tap below the knee and test our reflexes, and we'd all shriek with laughter as our lower legs shot up. I was about nine when I asked her, 'Will I always have skinned knees?' The scabs and abrasions came from climbing trees and falling off roller skates and my bicycle. No, she assured me. I was about 16 when I asked her, 'When you are out on a date, and a boy puts his hand on your knee, what does it mean?' More important, she responded, how does it make you feel? Uncomfortable, I replied. Then tell him to move his hand. It's your knee. You decide if he can put his hand there or not. We were on our knees every night around three sides of hers and Dad's bed saying the Rosary for seven years. The family that prays together stays together, she'd say. The seven years began after Dad's first suicide attempt. Mom wanted prayer to do what doctors had not been able to do – free him from sadness. The prayers ended when he closed the garage doors and started the car. She kept her hand on my knee during the entire 45-minute drive from the hospital to our home.

My mother sat erectly in the car, jaw set as she does when tragedy strikes as if her small frame and narrow shoulders would carry us all. Her presence, her touch, the shape of her body filled Carl, Pete and me, entering the spaces where courage and strength and hope were – before Sarah died.

In the hospital before my mother and brothers arrived, nature's cushion, shock, was buffering me since hospital personnel had not provided me an emotionally safe place to begin to grieve, a place so vital that without it grieving – that profound, necessary, complicated yet normal set of emotions – cannot begin. Without it, my mother tried to bury a lifetime of griefs. Grief will not remain buried, would that it were so. For my mother, the seemingly insurmountable mountain of grief, thought buried, erupted without warning throughout her life in the form of incapacitating depressions, evidence of the undone work of facing the sadness of newborn Robert's death, and Little Joe, and Joe's and my dad's suicides that occurred during an era that shunned the victims of suicide. She told me of spending hours in psychiatrists' and psychologists' offices just sitting. 'Would you like to talk about anything today?' a doctor would ask her. No, thank you, she'd respond or she'd just shake her head slightly, moving it from one side to the other. And a cup of sand would be thrown on the bubbling volcanoes. In the months after Sarah died, she would give me something she could not give herself, the most life-affirming, life-sustaining gift anyone can give another person – a safe place to grieve. And I have never figured out how she could give what she did not have. She was my optimist when in grief I saw only despair. She held me so close that I thought she was breathing for me when I thought I had stopped doing so. She prodded me to stop feeling sorry for myself, to do something for someone else when wallowing threatened to become my new way of life. She laughed when, without Sarah, the world was devoid of humor. I'd glare at her, and she'd tell another joke, padding her gift, my safe place, with her own armor, her own special stamp. Because of her gift, I hold my friends and family members when they are hurting; I hold them as if I might never be able to again because I know now that there is no promise of tomorrow; our loved ones can be taken from us at any time and without warning. The despair that loss brings is the black hole of grief and the only light, the only way out, is through my mother's gift.

The tires crunched over the gravel in our driveway as Carl eased the car to a stop, and I noticed that our lawn, our house, the trees that lined the driveway were all gray. Glennie Rhodes was in the front yard. She was crying when she came to the door of the car and said through the open window, 'I wanted this baby.' She mashed wads of Kleenex between her clenched fingers. Her face was blotchy red for an instant until she and it were consumed by fog. 'I'll come and cry with you,' I heard her say before her words faded.

Tom's shoulders slumped as he stood in the driveway flanked by Molly and Emily. He opened the car door for me and put his arm around my shoulders and willed me to walk up the front steps. We crossed the front porch and went into the house while my mother and brothers watched the girls outside. He sat on the couch by the window that let in gray light. I heard him say something, but I couldn't understand his words; he was crying. I put my arms around his body that I couldn't see through the haze or feel because I didn't have any skin on.

That's how the girls found us when they would no longer be restrained outside with my mother, Carl, and Pete. They ran into the house to get answers to unanswerable questions, for logic where there was none.

Molly was saying something. I had to concentrate so that I could understand her.

'She couldn't,' Tom was saying.

'I couldn't what?' I asked him.

Then Emily was talking.

'Yes,' Tom told her.

'Yes to what?' I asked him.

'Why do I have to stay outside with Grammie?' Emily asked.

'You didn't let me hold her,' Molly said.

'She couldn't,' Tom said.

'I want to see her,' Molly said. 'I want to see Sarah. When can I see her? You got to hold her for two hours.' Molly stomped her once red, now gray-leather shoes on the carpet.

Molly wants to see Sarah. How can I take her to see Sarah? What will she look like? I was eight, a year older than Molly, when I stood in the dining room and gazed at the picture of Robert that my father had someone at the funeral home take. That life-sized picture was more like an oil painting or a pastel than a photograph for its muted colors, and it was the only vision my mother and us kids had of Robert. His skin looked pasty, powdered, the color of biscuit dough. His lips were lipstick-red, too red to be a real baby's lip color. He looked more like a not very good-looking doll than a baby brother. When Little Joe died, I was four, a year younger than Em. I don't remember his dead face, though I was at the funeral and the casket was open during the graveside service. I remember what he wore. And I keep a picture of him in my mind because he was the most beautiful of all of us. He had our Dad's black hair and olive skin and dark alert eyes and a bud of his Roman nose. Maybe I don't remember Little Joe's dead face because I didn't look. If Molly looks I should be with her, but I don't want to see Sarah again. If Molly cries how could I comfort her? I have nothing left to give. Oh, my God, please help me, I prayed. In an instant I knew to call our regular pediatrician.

'I need,' someone said. 'It's in your bedroom. Please.'

Get something for someone from my bedroom. Oh, sure, I heard myself saying. I walked toward the bedroom until I remembered that Sarah's cradle was in the bedroom, and I couldn't walk anymore. I turned back toward the hazy gray living room that was filling with people and noise like surging mumble. 'I can't . . . her cradle.'

My mother's arm was around my shoulders.

A phone was ringing a muffled ring. Car doors shut as if they closed on pillows. Daisy howled in the backyard as if to sound an alarm that nothing was right.

'T,' Tom was saying, 'It's Kath on the phone. She wants to talk to you.'

'I can't talk on the phone.'

'Can she and Glenda come over?'

'No.' I was afraid to face my closest friends, afraid to face the joy we had shared these past months anticipating this baby, afraid to face the sorrow with them.

'Please come tomorrow after we get back from the funeral home. About 11,' Tom said into the phone.

The phone rang again. 'Mom and Dad are coming for Molly and Emily's ballet recital next month,' Tom said. 'Have their yellow mums arrived?'

'I don't know what you are saying. I don't know anything about mums,' I told him. I found the mums and weeks later I planted them on Glennie Rhodes' side of the house. For years after they bloomed brilliant, big, lemon-yellow blossoms. They were blooming when we sold the house and moved to a bigger one. The house held happy memories and sad ones, but it was the mums I focused on the last time we backed out of the driveway.

Pat Borton, a neighbor and friend, arrived holding a tray of ham and cheese slices. Pat's two daughters, Anita and Diana, and Molly and Emily played together. On weekends when Tom was home and not on fire duty, I'd call Pat to see if it was convenient for the girls to visit. If she said yes, I'd walk to the edge of our driveway and Molly and Em would walk by themselves the short block to the Borton's house. Pat would be outside watching the girls skip or run toward her. Once she waved that she was on duty and I'd sent a thank-you-wave back, Tom and I knew we'd have at least an hour to ourselves. Before I could get back inside the house, I'd find Tom already in bed waiting for me. Months earlier, Pat told me that her nephew had died of sudden infant death syndrome. We both cried, and I crossed my arms over my pregnant womb and vowed I would keep this baby safe.

Night came and all the grays turned to blacks.

My mother said she had to go home.

'No,' I protested.

'It's late. I'll be here first thing in the morning. Can you sleep?'

'Sleep? Oh, no.'

'Try.'

She held me close and long.

'I love you,' my mother said. 'I'll see you for breakfast. First thing in the morning, I'll be here. Molly and Emily have eaten dinner. The refrigerator is full of food. So many people have brought things. The girls have brushed their teeth and had their baths. No school tomorrow. Try to sleep.'

There was nothing more when she left. There was only black and empty. Carl and Pete left with her. Tom held my hand. His skin on my hand felt warm and good. Nothing else was.

8. The rhythm of sleep breathing

Tom's breathing was steady, full, relaxed. My breaths were hesitant, shallow, torturous. His rhythm was to the count of four . . . in, two, three, four, out, two, three, four. I could only hold to the count of three if I concentrated. When I stopped thinking about the counts, I had no beat, no rhythm. My breathing was erratic, forced, and painful. The digital clock's large red numbers glared: 12.52, 12.57, 1.00, 1.06.

He began to breathe more deeply. If he were to fall asleep before I did, I could not even try to match the slow rhythm of sleep breathing. He would be asleep, and I would be awake alone. I moved closer to his body. His back was toward me. My knees fit inside his, spoon-like. The cavity made by my empty womb was filled by his buttocks. I brought my left arm across his chest and rested my right arm on top of his, matching its curled shape. It was easier to try to match the rhythm of his breathing while pressed against him.

In, two, three, four, five, out, two, three, four, five. Again, again. Still I could only hold to three. His breathing was slower, deeper. He was falling asleep. If he fell asleep, I wondered if I could breathe at all. I took in air, a quiet sob, as my bottom lip trembled. Tom turned over, faced me and wrapped his arms around me. His hands moved over my back, slowly, warmly, smoothly. Everywhere he touched me the skin on his hands covered my skinless back, over and over. I held on, I could breathe without having to concentrate. I held on for warmth, for breath, for life: tighter, closer, warmer. His lips caressed my hair, my cheeks, my eyelids, my neck. He moaned softly. In a minute he was asleep. I gasped for breath.

9. Time to scream

'The service will be private,' I told the woman sitting next to me who had introduced herself as Elizabeth, 'so there is no need to put the time in the newspaper.' We sat in burgundy colored, straight-backed leather chairs identical to 30 others in the room at the funeral home. My eyes studied the shiny brass upholstery tacks that attached the leather to the wood-frame of the chair. I wanted to find a tack missing. I studied each chair that lined the walls and each chair placed around the table. Row after row, chair after chair, I focused on every shiny brass tack in the spacious room. All the tacks were neatly in place. There weren't any empty places.

The empty chairs were in the room as if waiting for people to come, to fill them up and talk about burying the person who has made their lives empty. 'What's a hole for?' my mother asked each of us when we were four years old.

'To sew up,' I told her.

'If Treesa doesn't think she did it then I guess I did,' said Mike, thinking Mom was accusing him of breaking something.

'To put things in,' said Joe.

'To dig in,' said Carl.

'For burying treasure,' said Frank.

'To look into,' said Pete.

Three chairs on the other side of the massive table were occupied by Tom and two men from the funeral home. Elizabeth and I sat across from them. The wide rectangular table stretched between us in an empty gulf, intensifying the light and dark chocolate hues of the walnut grain. Light and dark, full and empty, night and day, pain and joy, skin and no skin. My eyes began to sting so I looked down at the rug. It was oriental and thick, red mostly, blood red.

'Is Sarah spelled with or without an H?' Elizabeth asked.

'With an H, and have the papers say that Sarah was "the new-born daughter" of Mr and Mrs Vigour. Some people don't know that I had the baby.'

'What about the name of the minister?' Elizabeth asked.

'I'll have to call you after I find out who it will be.' What I meant was, I'll call you after I find one. Although I was raised Catholic, I hadn't been to church in years. I didn't have a priest to bury our baby. And I was not going to be a foxhole Catholic who would call a priest only when I needed one. But experience brings us to religion, one priest had said years ago when I was still attending church and listening to sermons.

'Can you arrange to pick up the baby from the hospital after the doctors finish the autopsy?' I asked Elizabeth. I couldn't say body. Elizabeth nodded as if baby was the right word to use.

Across the table, Tom was talking to a man about kinds of caskets. He asked my opinion of a casket style or color or something about brass handles versus wood. I told him I liked his choice, although I don't know what he asked me. Being in that room and discussing Sarah's funeral was not real to me. I wanted to go home, to be with Molly and Emily. I wanted everything to go back to normal.

I handed Elizabeth the gown that Molly and Emily had worn when I brought them home from the hospital. It was light yellow and printed with darker yellow ducks. The gown had a drawstring at the bottom, and the sleeves had extra pieces of material to fold over the baby's hands so she wouldn't scratch herself with her fingernails. My mother had given me the gown and a matching blanket before Molly was born. She wore it home from the hospital seven years ago, then Emily wore it two years later. Now it would be Sarah's always.

The blanket that matched the gown was dingy-gray now, and its edges were frayed from too much loving. This was the blanket Molly named Acey when she was 18 months old and distraught because she'd lost it. She followed me in and out of rooms in the house as we looked for her blanket. Her anguish seemed to ease when I chattered. So I held her hand and asked, "Where's Molly's blanket? Where's Molly's blanket?" as we went from the kitchen to the living room to the bathroom.

'Uun no,' she answered in language I understood. I don't know, she responded to me again and again. Then I opened the door to her bedroom. There on the floor was the blanket. Delighted, I shouted, 'I see it.' For Molly, the joy in my voice merged with the comforting sight of her blanket. The words *I see it* were forever after words of happiness, reunion, security. So Acey came to be.

She took Acey everywhere with her. She dragged it through sand and waves at the ocean. She took it to nursery school where it hung on her peg with her coat until it was time to come home. It went to birthday parties when she was two, three, and four years old. By the time she was five, the blanket no longer traveled with her – it stayed home to be comfort at night. Affection for the ragged blanket permitted passage from infancy's dependence to a lifetime of independence.

Emily wore the yellow gown with the yellow ducks when I brought her home from the hospital, but she was not wrapped in Acey. Molly would not have parted with it, and I wouldn't have asked her to. And Acey was too worn to wrap around a new baby to bring her home from the hospital. Emily didn't need a blanket as it was a warm day in spring. Chrysanthemums, red buds, dogwood blossoms had burst out in joyous celebration of her life. It was warm, too, the day I came home from the hospital without Sarah. She wouldn't have needed the blanket either.

'Do you have a blanket that I can wrap the baby in?' Elizabeth was asking.

'No, not one that matches.' I reached into my wallet to get a five-dollar bill. I started to hand it to Elizabeth. I was going to ask her to find a blanket to match the yellow in the gown. Then I remembered that it didn't matter about the blanket because the casket would be closed, so I told Elizabeth that we wouldn't need a blanket.

Molly wanted desperately to see the new baby. The night before coming to the funeral home, I called our regular pediatrician. If I woke him, he didn't tell me. I can hear the softness of his voice even now, years after that conversation.

'The children will be expecting to see a Gerber Baby,' the doctor said. 'They won't see that.'

What would make Sarah look less like a Gerber Baby, the autopsy or just death itself, I wondered while the doctor was on the phone. Maybe death alone was reason enough not to look. But death can't be hidden from our girls. Her death was permeating everything for all of us. I couldn't research it all then – all the questions that needed answers, that must be answered. Should they look at Sarah? How do I explain the scars where doctors cut open her head to look at her brain? She was so pink and warm. What color is death's face when it isn't powdered like Robert's? Would her forehead be permanently wrinkled from the pain she must have endured before she died? So many questions went unsaid when I asked, 'Doctor, Molly is begging me to let her see the baby. And then there is Emily. She would come, too, if we went to see the baby. What would you do?'

He and I had been through cuts that needed stitches. His stitches were neat and his voice was calm and nonjudgmental. He never asked me how I let an accident happen. Even on the day Molly and Emily found a jar of Sudafed tablets in my purse and ate several of the pretty red pills that looked just like candy red hots. They chewed pills while I vacuumed unaware. He treated the girls and me during that emergency room visit. He had the girls vomit a total of seven pills, and he told me to sit down. After I did, he said I was about to faint. Fear and relief drained my face of its color and my body of its ability to remain upright. The mutual trust between us was built upon years of discussing treatment and respecting each other's area of expertise. His decisions had been valid. This call was his, right or wrong. What we would see and what we wouldn't see during those next few days would haunt each of us for the rest of our lives.

The doctor spoke tenderly, softly, yet deliberately. He must have known that I would hear his words always. My friend, the pediatrician, said, 'Keep the casket closed.'

'Good night,' I said.

A man came into the room and whispered to Elizabeth. She nodded to him and said softly to me, 'A call for you. This man will take you to the phone.'

I assumed that Molly or Emily was calling. We had been gone for more than an hour. But instead of a little voice saying, 'When are you coming home, Mommy?' the neonatologist's anxious voice said, 'You cannot have an autopsy done. You cannot afford it.' At first feeling assaulted, my stomach tightened, then loosened when I became indignant. Then, realizing he had no say, no input into this decision, I was in control.

'I'm having it done,' I told him.

'I don't advise it.'

'I'm not asking for your advice.' I said and hung up the phone.

I went back to the room where Tom was and Elizabeth and the two other men from the funeral home. Tom was moving toward the front door.

Driving home, I told him about the call from the doctor. 'It's none of his business whether or not we have an autopsy,' he said. 'He's got a hell of a nerve calling us at the funeral home. The decision is already made. And asking for you instead of me. Does he think he can bully you?'

The doctor knew nothing of our finances or my recent inheritance from my grandmother. His reasoning did not make sense.

Nothing about our home was familiar. Walking up the steps to the front porch, I heard a low awkward humming. Inside, people in an unfamiliar situation didn't know whether to try to make jokes or smile at an acquaintance or just concentrate on feeling droplets of sweat run behind their ears and between their shoulder blades. Human shapes moved throughout the living room in ripples. I couldn't focus on faces. The moving blur was like looking at an anthill from a few feet away: I know there are individual ants, yet I just see the mound move. Foresters were there from the Weyerhaeuser paper mill where Tom worked, and government foresters, foresters' wives, and teachers from the elementary school where I worked. My shoulders bumped other people's shoulders. Hugs and muffled I'm sorrys, came from all directions. I smelled the perfume of shirts just out of the dryer or just off the clothesline or jackets just back from the cleaners. I felt out of place in my red-and-white-checked maternity dress that had wrinkled when I folded my arms tightly across my empty womb, yet each of us in that room was out of place.

Then out of the hum and blur, Kath and Glenda's faces emerged. I found their hands and pulled them toward the kitchen. Kath is Molly's godmother. Glenda was my boss at the elementary school where all our children went. She was the teacher; I was her aide. Together we taught 26 kindergarteners whatever they were capable of learning: some learned how to read and some never learned to sit still. Teaching came naturally to her, suited her. She was teaching me how to teach almost without my knowing it. How important those two women had become to me; for years we'd depended on each other as we hadn't had family around. Mom and Carl and Pete had moved to our East Coast town only recently. Glenda, Kath, and I had not spoken in the past four life-changing days, then I remembered I hadn't told them about the baby's birth.

'Come to the kitchen right now, you two. I'll pour the coffee. It was the oddest delivery. I have to tell you.'

I forgot. In that instant, in the company of my friends, I forgot. In my desire to tell them about the baby's birth just as they had shared their birth experiences with me – I forgot that Sarah had died. During the delivery I was only thinking of the baby to come. I had no thoughts of any other outcome. It was that joy, that expectation that I wanted to share with my close friends. I smiled. I laughed. I told them what happened until I remembered.

When I did, the pain came in a fresh rush as if she had just died. I never forgot again.

We sat on bar stools and rested our elbows on the counter where, for years, we had traded recipes, discussed children's discipline problems, explored our newly evolving roles as wives and mothers, tried to imagine that we were making something of ourselves in the early years of women's liberation – the 70s and 80s – even though our days were spent changing diapers and enduring two-year-olds' temper tantrums. I told them about the contractions being mild, so mild that I could not believe it when the nurse said it was time to push. But something happened. Each time I tried to push, the pain was terrific. It wasn't like the other deliveries. Pushing for the others was not painful. I pleaded with the nurse-midwife to do something, but she told me to keep pushing and said how wonderful it was that the baby was small. I wasn't tearing and wouldn't need an episiotomy. 'If the baby was small, why did it feel as if it were coming out sideways?' I asked them.

Kath was laughing, pretending not to take me seriously, but actually, she knew that Glenda and I remembered the episiotomy was worse for her than any other part of labor and delivery.

'No laughing,' I told her challenging her, baiting her.

She bit. 'You earth mother,' she said. 'If you wouldn't be such a hero and take some Demerol or have a caudal, you wouldn't get yourself into these situations.'

'All right,' I agreed, 'but remember, Kath, you couldn't raise your head off the pillow for 12 hours because of the medicine you took. Remember the doctor said you'd have a headache to end all headaches if you did? And, Glenda, you went to the hospital after lunch, and you didn't see Scott until the next day when you woke up. I wanted to see the baby right away.'

'Pain was the price you paid,' Kath said.

I knew she was right, but I said, 'Well, it didn't hurt until it was time to push.'

'Then it was too late for pain medicine,' said Glenda.

'All the Lamaze literature says it's not supposed to hurt when you get to the pushing part. It hadn't hurt for Molly and Em,' I said.

'Naaaah,' they said in unison.

'How would you two know? By the time you got to the pushing part, you'd already had medicine,' I said.

'It wasn't the time for me to test some man's theory about how to have a baby,' Glenda said.

'There are times to cover your you-know-what, and this is one of them,' Kath said.

'It's a good thing I'm not looking for sympathy from you two,' I said laughing. 'And, remember, you're drinking my coffee.'

'Okay, so tell us what happened,' Glenda said.

'Well, Tom said I bent the bed frame. I reached under the mattress, found some springs and metal strips and squeezed. He said the bed frame was bent after I let go. But before I did let go, I heard the baby cry. Tom said we had another girl. And the nurse-midwife was so excited she screamed, "Apgar Score 10".'

'They wrapped her in a blue and yellow blanket and handed her to me. I'll tell you something: I was mad at her then. But only for a second or so . . . well, a few minutes maybe. God, that was a painful delivery. I unwrapped her; she was beautiful. The cheesy skin coating was in the folds of her neck and under her arms and behind her knees. As I looked under each arm and leg and counted her fingers and toes, she seemed like a tired rag doll. I guess the others were like rag dolls just after birth, but this baby seemed more tired. Maybe the delivery was hard on her too. Then I started to feel sorry for her. I wrapped her up again and held her close to me. My heart was beating so hard that I thought it would beat its way out of my chest. I brought her closer to me. She found the nipple and fell asleep. That was the last time I held her.'

They started to cry before I did. They remembered before I did. I heaved, inhaling the horror of Sarah's death. As if to shield myself from the intake, I covered my face with my hands and sobbed. Kath and Glenda's arms squeezed my shoulders.

'When is the funeral?' Glenda asked. 'We'll be there with you.'

'It's private. It will be just the family.'

'Well, we'll see you after. Call me. I don't have to work Wednesday. I'll be home,' Kath said.

'Call me in the middle of the night if you want to,' Glenda said as she and Kath left the kitchen and made their way through the crowd in the living room so they could leave by the front door.

The phone rang. It was my friend, Vera. I never have to wonder what Vera is thinking. She tells me. Once I became accustomed to her, I found myself being honest – completely honest with her and myself. Kath and Glenda and I, on the other hand, alter the truth a bit to avoid hurting each other. We dance around each other's feelings. We're all a good bit Irish. 'Someone's at my door, I'll call you later,' might really mean: 'I have been on this phone for 20 minutes listening to you fuss about how your husband hasn't repaired the screen in the back door. I'm tired of listening, and besides, I have to do laundry this morning.' Or, if one of us is bothered by something and not volunteering what it is, the other two of us might wonder and hint, but we dare not ask for fear of intruding. Not Vera.

'When's the funeral?'

'It's private, Vera. Just family.'

'That's not what I asked you. When's the funeral?'

'No, Vera, I mean it. It's private.'

'There are times when your dear friends know how to help. You shouldn't have to do this alone.'

'No, Vera.'

'Why?'

'Because.'

'Because why?'

I turned my back to the people in the kitchen, and I cupped the mouthpiece of the phone with my hand. In a low voice I said, 'Vera, I think I'll scream. I can't believe I'm having Sarah's funeral. If I start screaming, I won't be able to stop. I don't want anyone to hear me.'

'I'll come for the girls first thing in the morning. They can play with Jena while you are at the funeral.'

'Thanks, Vera, but we need to do this as a family. We all need to say goodbye. I was at one of my brother's funerals when I was four. On this, I know what I'm doing.'

'I'll see you after. I love you.'

Love was as tangible as the Saran wrapped tray of sliced roast beef and cheese, or the envelope full of $320 in small bills – the overflow from the flower fund collected at Tom's office. Love came in hugs that gathered the pieces of our shattered souls. It came with pretty bows from florists as well as from the reddened eyes of friends saying the seemingly lame, yet compassionately comforting, 'I don't know what to say.'

Forever after I would know the need to go quickly to loved ones in pain. How lopsided, I used to think, that the new griever is flooded with sympathizers at first and then endures months of a drought of visitors. Rather, the time of public mourning is immediately after death. Grievers can draw on that love, either literally or by calling up the memories, in the months and years of private grieving.

10. The rosebud

When I woke up the next day, the morning of Sarah's funeral, the warm, sunny weather seemed out of sync with the event before us. How could the sun light the bedroom? Where were the black clouds? And rain so cold and blowing it stings stockinged legs? And wind that threatens hurricanes?

I closed my eyes and pulled the sheet over my shoulders. Maybe it isn't so . . . Sarah . . . the sun. But my closed eyes saw Sarah's pudgy cheeks, her hair the color of mahogany, her pink lips, her slate-black eyes rimmed with the promise of becoming blue.

The night before I had told my mother that the thought of seeing the casket being lowered into the grave was ungluing me, she assured me it would remain above ground until we left. In mentally previewing the emotionally necessary, symbolic ritual of burying Sarah – all I could focus on was watching the grave workers feeding, hand over hand, more and more of the supporting strap as the casket slipped below the level of the ground. I cried thinking about it as I had cried 16 years earlier thinking of my dad's handsome, athletic body decaying.

The house was quiet with Tom and the girls still asleep, an eerie quiet after being filled for two days with mourners. The perfume of flowers wafted from the living room to the bedrooms, along with their airborne pollens, allergens, irritants. Our normal slightly unkempt house with its clutter – magazines on the coffee table or on the arm of a chair, newspapers on the sofa, teddy bears and dolls in strollers or baby beds, books, mail on the mantel or on top of the piano, crayons, magic markers, shoes – was too neat. As I surveyed the living room and turned to go to the bathroom, my bare feet left imprints in the springy pile of newly vacuumed carpet. Even the house was changed by death.

I rotated the faucet in the bathtub all the way to hot and cupped the cold water until it began to warm my hand; I pulled the lever diverting the flow from the tub to the shower and stepped in. At once, the warm water activated the letdown reflex and Sarah's milk dripped from my breasts. My shoulders shook, my eyes stung. I couldn't feel my hot tears because they were washed away by the shower's spray. Lochia, the bleeding after childbirth, ran down my legs and swirled in red pools around my feet and between my toes before disappearing down the drain. I got out of the shower quickly, so I didn't have to see any more reminders of childbirth, didn't have to watch any more of me go down the drain.

My navy blue maternity dress with small red and pink flowers was on Sarah's changing table where I'd laid it the night before, along with a nursing bra and thick support stockings. Soon, my legs would stop aching, and I could stop wearing the stockings. But it would be weeks before regular clothes would fit. My eyes drifted from my clothes to the empty changing table, the empty bins. Just the day before the bins were filled with the miniature undershirts, the gowns in pinks, yellows, and greens with matching receiving blankets soft as cat's fur, one-piece play outfits, the diapers my teachers at school had given me at a surprise shower, the baby wipes and Desitin for diaper rash, the jars of Q-tips, diaper pins, cotton balls, the towels and wash cloths, the dresses in sizes 0–3 months that had been Sarah's older sisters', the matching tights and socks, baby rattles. My mother was in the living room when Molly asked for a big safety pin, and I headed, without thinking, to Sarah's changing table for a diaper pin until I remembered that Sarah wouldn't be coming home. Without my willing it, I heard myself inhale as if I were trying to take in a reality that was new again, fresh as the moment I learned she had died. My mother must have gathered Sarah's baby clothes and dipes and wipes and rattles. So the changing table was empty, looking as it had a month ago, before the girls and I had gone to the attic to find the box marked 'infant clothes,' before we'd washed, dried, and folded each tiny shirt, each little gown. The remembering made it new again. I gasped, waking Tom.

'What time is it?' he asked.

'Eight ten.'

'Are the girls awake?'

'I don't think so.'

'How are you?'

'Drained.'

'Can you manage?'

'Like having my legs amputated. It will be over. I won't have to dread it anymore.'

Tom noticed my shoulders slump, defeated. He followed my eyes as they stared at each empty bin of the changing table, and as they stopped moving to focus on nothing. He wanted to get my attention, to bring me back to the morning tasks of feeding and dressing the girls, so he hugged me. When my heavy arms would not raise to hug back, he knew I was somewhere else, as distant to him as if in another century. He pulled on a pair of shorts and a T-shirt; he'd put on his suit after fixing breakfast and getting the girls dressed.

From our home the cemetery was a 15-minute drive.

'It's 20 minutes until ten. We'll be late,' Tom said, issuing his last call for us to get into the car.

'They won't start without us,' I told him.

In my arms I clutched my purse and two cold, unopened bottles of beer.

'It's time to go,' Tom called. I didn't see the girls; I guessed they were already in the car. I hadn't seen or heard them all morning.

I was swept to the already opened front door by a sense of obligation. Something in my genes or upbringing said, you can't not go. I always finish everything on my plate, always drink the last of my milk. I could not have told my legs to move me through the front door, but I felt myself stumbling toward the car. The front door to the passenger seat was open. I sat in the seat and slid the beers, my props, into the side-door pocket of the Volvo wagon. I had no tranquilizers, no sleeping pills, no sleep, no skin. If I screamed or felt like it, I would drink the beers.

Molly and Emily were in the back seat already buckled in. Emily squeezed several folds of her security blanket into her left hand and sucked the thumb of her right hand and gazed at the window. Until that morning, Molly had been leaving her blanket at home, but she held hers tightly and she, too, fingered one of its corners and sucked her thumb. Normally the car would be filled with their chatter and Tom's and my responses, but tension manifested in silence.

Many cars and trucks lined the narrow winding asphalt paths of Green Leaf Cemetery. Since ours was a private family service for the four of us and my mother and my brothers, I thought there must have been services for someone else going on at the same time. One parking place was left. It was directly in front of the funeral home's green tent. I thought there was not enough room for our car. We should find someplace else to park, maybe at the end of the line of vehicles, a quarter of a mile ahead. Walking back would delay the starting for at least ten minutes, mercifully. Before I told Tom what I was thinking, he parked the car in the space that was too small.

I shut the car door and turned toward the funeral home's green tent a few yards away when the weight of my empty arms pulled me down. An eroding slope of sandy dirt and pebbles and sparsely distributed blades of grass and clumps of moss rushed toward me. Before I hit it or it hit me, I surveyed the gravesite and saw three faces I recognized: Jamie King who taught me biology, anatomy and physiology, and genetics, and moored his cat-rigged boat at the sailing club. But this was a family-only service. Next to Jamie was Calvin Stokes, my principal, my friend, my boss, and next to him was Annette Angst, who had made beef stew elegant when she served it at a baby shower for me before Emily was born. I couldn't make eye contact so I looked down at their shoes: Jamies' brown deck shoes, Mr Stokes' wingtips, and Annette's shiny patent pumps, neat, pointed, proper, pretty, so like her. Beyond them were rows and rows of oxfords, loafers, work boots, dress flats, high heels. Pair after pair, two by two. Seeing the shoes of my friends made my arms not weigh so much. Could they have known I would have fallen without them? Because they were there, I could carry the heavy weight of my empty arms.

Four folding chairs were placed in front of the miniature white casket. I wished they weren't for us. No one should have to sit in them. Behind the casket stood Brother John, the Baptist preacher who would deliver the sermon. He rolled the stem of a rosebud between his thumb and forefinger. A rosebud, he said, has the potential to become a rose, yet it does not.

Brother John had called me the night before.

'Do you have someone for the services?'

The kindly man reminded me of Mr Rogers of *Mr Rogers' Neighborhood*. He wore blue canvas lace-up shoes and spoke slowly, softly. He ran the vacation Bible school every summer for children of any or no religion. Molly and Emily wanted to become Baptists after one week of making papier-mâché crosses and coloring cutout pictures of the apostles.

'Would you handle the service, Brother John?'

'Of course.'

At that moment I thought of becoming a Baptist, too. How had I stopped attending Mass? A habit as much a part of my life as eating breakfast. Was it the church's ruling on birth control?

'The pope's gone too far when he enters my bedroom,' my friend Kath told me when I asked her how we could think of taking the pill and Communion.

'It's one or the other, Kath.'

'If you believe the pope has a place in your bedroom,' she said.

A lifelong habit ended, I thought for only a short time, when I couldn't concentrate on the Mass while shushing two noisy, wiggly toddlers. I kept saying I'd start back and hadn't, so I was in a town where I had no connection to the local Catholic church, and after a trouble-free pregnancy, Tom and I had to plan a funeral. Since attending church wasn't Tom's thing, it became mine. The thought of introducing myself to a priest and saying I was a Catholic once, and asking him to come to the gravesite and say a few words to comfort a family he didn't know paralyzed me. Maybe my Irish guilt held me back, maybe shock. So, when a Baptist friend had called last night and asked if we had someone for the services and I said, no, and she asked if we would like her to call Brother John. Then he called me.

The pastor's words, delivered in his mellow, soothing voice, contrasted with the harsh reminder of the purpose of the gathering, so I listened to the sounds and not the words. I drifted mentally, almost floated, out of the group of mourners toward the billowing clouds suspended in the blue sky. I looked back from my vantage point in the clouds and saw myself, a 32-year-old with short brown hair that frizzes on humid days, with arms and legs covered in freckles, sitting in the beige metal folding chair atop an emerald green mat that resembled grass only in its placement. I was startled by this view of myself because what didn't show was the devastation. My gut churned and rippled; my thoughts raced uncontrollably. I looked as if I had slept and eaten in the past four days, though I hadn't. I looked as if I had skin on, but I was an open wound. I looked as if I were in control, but I didn't know if I would start screaming.

Tom was next to me wearing a white, permanent press, dress shirt that had come from the back of the closet and showed the characteristic wrinkles of having been shoved and crowded for too long. He hated wearing ties; he said they made his neck itch, but the two, pointed, blue-stripped panels hung from his neck. He had on his suit pants.

The dress Molly wore had been plucked from the pile of clean clothes, unironed. The strands of her hair that had not made it into her ponytail lifted and fell with the light breezes. She was on the other side of me in my mother's lap sucking her thumb. My mother, all 100 lbs of her, looked like a giant in a floor-length beige dress with small orange flowers because her strength showed in the set of her shoulders. Emily sat in my lap and occasionally kicked her feet, making a popping sound because her too-loosely-buckled shoes flapped.

To the right of the casket and dominating the landscape was a horseshoe-shaped piece of Styrofoam covered with hundreds of pink rosebuds sent by our sailing friends, Barbara and Preston Sellers. The curved shape and the blends of dusty pinks were a blur until I focused on one rosebud. Its small perfectly formed petals were made of a soft pile, like velvet, in shades of pink that ranged from a pale blush to a rich Windsor rose. The rosebud itself was exquisite but was even more wondrous for the unfolding it promised. Like a baby. My eyes stung and the rosebud blurred. There were other flowers on stands – funeral sprays. Whites and pinks with babies' breath and ribbons. Flowers and more flowers.

Holding Little Joe during the year and a half that he lived, my mother's face would be so full of happiness that her cheeks pushed her eyes into slits, and her mouth opened so wide that when her laughter came out it filled the room as he played with her red curls and tried to put his fingers in her mouth. I remember the sounds of his giggles. I remember him vomiting, turning blue, gasping for breath, and my mother's face collapsing and sinking in, and the laughter stopped. I grew up learning the meanings of the words *blue baby* and *congenital heart trouble*.

Behind the flowers, pine trees lined the outer edges of Green Leaf Cemetery. When I smell pine needles or hear Caribbean accents, I am four. I am walking with Christine to the blueberry field behind my grandparents' summer home, Wabeno, in Lake Placid, New York. Christine is from the Dominican Republic. I am so happy being with her that unexpectedly tears of joy and reunion filled my eyes decades later when I visited the Caribbean and heard the people speaking in her voice. Gathering blueberries with Christine may have been the only time that summer that I wasn't surrounded by my family's grief. We were visiting my grandparents in Lake Placid when Little Joe died.

The only light that shone into my crib at Wabeno came from the bedroom's open door. My mother was standing in the doorway. The light from the hallway behind her made her dress appear to billow and float. I couldn't see her face. I heard her voice. 'Little Joe is sick. Daddy and I are taking him to the hospital . . . Yes, I will fill your bottle.' I was drinking chocolate milk when I heard the front door slam.

Tufted pale blue satin lined the tiny casket and cushioned Little Joe, pillow-like. He wore the red and black plaid shorts with straps that went over his shoulders and crossed in back and the white shirt with an appliqué of a Scottie dog in the same red and black plaid as the shorts. The dog had a black beret. It is the same outfit he wore on Sunday mornings, and the time he pulled himself to a standing position by grabbing handfuls of the flowery-red slipcover on the chair in the living room. I put a baby bottle full of milk and a blanket into the casket and stepped back to look at the grassy valley amid outcroppings of the flat blue-tinted rock of the Adirondack Mountains, unaware I was committing the moment to memory. Rain fell ever so slightly as the priest stopped speaking. Dad put his arm around Mom and whispered, 'See, Miz, even the heavens are crying.'

My brother Robert died three years later at birth. Just Dad went to the funeral. Mom was in the hospital recovering from the flu, and Mike and I and our new two-year-old-brother, Joe, stayed home with our housekeeper, babysitter, cook, Mildred. I remember crying when I heard that Robert had died. I must have sensed my mother's excitement in the months before he was born as her pregnancy progressed. I must have been grieving for joy that didn't come. He wore a white gown long enough to cover his feet and keep on going. The lace edging at the hem matched the lace on his cap that circled his face. Satin ribbons under his chin were tied in a bow and rested lightly on the gown's lace bodice. His face was a powdery white; his mouth was lipsticked red.

Our home was filled with flowers when I was 16; I could smell them before I opened the front door. My brothers Joe, Carl, Frank, Pete, and I had gone to our cottage on the Chesapeake Bay for a last week of swimming and sailing before the end of summer and the start of school. Our brother Mike stayed home with our parents. Our mother called to tell us to come home early because our father was dead.

Arrangements of flowers nearly as tall as I was lined the baseboards in the living room, dining room, and our parents' bedroom. Daisies in small glass vases and philodendrons in ceramic bowls were on the mantel piece; roses, prayer plants, and peace lilies were on the fireplace hearth; lily of the valley, bromeliads, and spider plants were on the coffee table in the living room; spiky, fuzzy cactuses and vases of cut flowers were on the piano; tulips, ferns and weeping figs, hyacinths, and palms were on the dining room table. It wasn't our home anymore; it belonged to flowers and death.

'Why do people bring flowers?' I asked my mother that day.

'They want to do something. They know we are hurting.'

Carol Talbot, my friend since childhood, sent Molly and Emily a box of chocolates that arrived the day before Sarah's funeral. The girls were enjoying selecting one each of the big pastel-colored candies after every meal, breakfast included. It was out of character for me to allow candy after breakfast, but I figured they needed any treat they could get. Carol was with me the day I had flowers instead of a father. She knows that flowers make my eyes itch, my nose run, my head throb, my body sneeze, and my heart ache.

The night before Sarah's funeral Brother John asked, 'What would you like me to say during the funeral?'

'Keep it short.'

'I mean, what would you like me to talk about?'

'I don't care. Just keep it short.'

Brother John mouthed words I did not hear. I watched him because if I looked anywhere else, my eyes saw the rosebuds or the casket between us. I hoped the woman from the funeral home, Elizabeth, had gotten a blanket. Sarah should have been wrapped in a blanket. I said it didn't matter when we were at the funeral home, but it does matter. The preacher's drone stopped. He placed the rosebud he'd been fingering on top of the casket. It was over. I didn't feel like screaming or crying. I didn't feel.

'If there is anything I can do for you, just let me know,' Calvin Stokes said.

'I want a job,' I told him.

'I mean it now, you just let me know what I can do for you,' he says.

'I mean it, Mr Stokes. I want a job.'

He nodded and left. What would I do if he didn't call? I couldn't stay home without Sarah. Soon Molly and Emily would be in school. Tom would go back to work. I couldn't be alone without Sarah.

'I'm so sorry,' someone said.

'I am too,' I said.

A teacher from school was crying. I put my arm around her shoulders and whispered in her ear, 'If you don't stop crying right now, I will start. And if I do, I assure you, we'll all drown.' She stopped crying and smiled. She gave me a teddy bear at the surprise baby shower at school. On a ruse of a teachers' meeting, I was summoned into the library after school one day. The library was full of large square boxes, all wrapped in pastel blues, pinks, lavenders, yellows. Each teacher had brought a box of paper diapers. Except the teacher who brought the fuzzy brown bear. The bear wore a T-shirt with letters saying: *Someone you love needs something to hug.*

I kept facing the people, so I couldn't see the casket behind me. I moved to the right side of the semicircle of people because it was farther from the casket. I embraced each person. I thanked each one for coming. Why would anyone want to come to such a sad event? I was grateful that they had. Maybe because they were there, I didn't feel like screaming. Talking to each person gave me something to do so I didn't have to think about why we were there. When I came to the end of the semicircle, I walked toward the car. I was afraid that if I waited any longer, the funeral home workers would begin lowering the casket, so I walked to the car and sat next to the still-cold beers and knew I had just done the most difficult thing I had ever had to do.

11. Arthritis and group B streptococcus

We hadn't expected Tom's family to come to the funeral. It was a seven-hour drive, and with few funerals in their family, attending them had not yet become their family's tradition. When each of Tom's grandparents died, his parents told us not come, that our obligations at home were more pressing. But it was to his family in Waynesboro, Virginia, his parents, his two brothers, his sister, and sister-in-law, that we escaped after we buried Sarah, to be embraced by other sets of arms, to be cared for, to leave our home, our place of mourning.

Against my protests, my mother thrust her most cherished possession into my arms as we pulled out of her driveway to head for Virginia. She, who had given up on organized religion, focused on reading the Bible. The church, she felt, had let her down after her prayers could not prevent my father's death and, again, after a priest came ostensibly to comfort our grieving, fatherless family and sexually molested my brother Mike, then 14. Solace for her came from reading her Bible. She would underline some passages and highlight others; she'd make notes in the margins, and tuck holy cards or birthday cards or hand written notes (hers or others') in between pages. It was a virtual scrapbook of her memories, aspirations, struggles, keepsakes. I was not a studier or even reader of the Bible, and knew I would not read hers, but she would hear none of it. I tucked her Bible between my seat and the car door.

We visited my friend Carol who lived then in nearby Nelson County, and I cried when it was time to leave, telling her that I didn't want to go back and face life at home without Sarah. She offered me her guest room. Stay a week or two, she said. My mouth dropped open at the possibility. A month, she added. And I've never loved her more or been more grateful for an invitation. For a moment, I thought about cool nights on her deck, watching the sun set behind the Appalachian Mountains, trading stories, drinking beer, rehashing our growing up years. Then I thought about Tom caring for the girls by himself and that I'd just be putting off grieving, and some part of me knew that I had to go home. I think I knew then that for emotional survival, I couldn't put off what was ahead, though I did not know and could not have predicted how difficult the next months or years would be, how much I would learn, and how I would be changed. I didn't stay with Carol for another reason: Tom. I'd followed him around like a lost puppy since Sarah; I couldn't watch him drive away.

It seemed like a little thing, to follow Tom and he to appreciate being needed, but it would have a big impact on our relationship. My gratitude for his being there for me when I was most needy would never end and would take trust to a new level. And years later, when his boss would close Tom's satellite office leaving him without a job, I experienced devastation from the other side. 'I can't think of anything to do,' he'd tell me in the weeks that followed. I'd stuffed my pockets with notes of jobs that needed doing just so that I could respond quickly. I'd turn so he couldn't see me pull out a note.

'How about changing the light bulb in the hall bathroom?'

'Good idea,' he'd say and head toward the cabinet where the light bulbs were stored.

After our five-day trip to Virginia, Tom went back to work and the girls went back to school. I wasn't ready yet to be by myself, so after I'd see them off, I'd go to my mother's house. On that first day back from Virginia, my mother asked me if I enjoyed reading her Bible. I don't remember how I answered, but I did go to the car to retrieve it, and it was not there. She loaned me what was her source of strength in tough times, and I lost it. I don't remember when or how, but it must have fallen out of the car because after a day or so of driving, I never saw it again. She didn't cry or yell at me; she just looked dumbfounded and never mentioned the loss again. After her death years later, my brothers and I were going through her things and found four Bibles with passages in each one underlined or highlighted. Cards and notes were tucked in between the pages. Four memory books: one for each of us.

On those days in May when I'd appear at her doorstep after taking the girls to school, she never seemed busy or acted as if she had other plans. She was always available. I would bring my box of stationery and address book and write thank you notes or letters to cousins who didn't know yet of the birth and death. Mom would sew. Often those visits, those healing visits, were wordless – like two soldiers who have returned from war, we didn't need to speak of what we'd experienced. I grew closer to her remembering snatches of days after Little Joe died when I was four, and my mother's only connection to life was the air she breathed, the rise and fall of her chest. She would have no energy or words or smiles. She would lie in bed and not hear me or see me though I stood by her side and talked to her or held her hand or stroked her arm. The house would be dark because my mother would not open the heavy red drapes printed with Egyptian figures that covered the picture windows in the living room, the ones that welcomed the morning sun, the ones that gave me a view of the world. In those days there was no world inside either, because my mother would not laugh or play the piano.

The drapes to my concern for Tom and our girls were drawn, too, much of the time, veiling them and their needs. I did not close them; they closed themselves. My mother and I could not have done otherwise. I understood her and myself in one epiphanic moment – a realization that freed us both of guilt and fault because breathing is all one can do sometimes. A death in the family makes each person needy, and a mother should nurture, especially then, but sometimes the drapes close, wrapping a mother in a much-needed cocoon so that she can emerge healed, stronger, enlightened.

When my mother opened the heavy red drapes, she would make pancakes shaped like Mickey Mouse's big ears and big head: three-in-one pancakes. She would read the comics to my brothers and me from *The Washington Post* which had four pages of daily comics. She read each comic strip. We listened to her every word while propped up by fluffed pillows leaned against the headboard of hers and Dad's bed. The bed was warm and soft and as inviting as she was on those days. We laughed.

Normally after school, Molly and Em would come to my room where I worked as a teacher's aide, but since I'd quit my job, I was in the pick-up line with the other mothers. The cars lined up one after the other, like adding beads to a necklace, on the shoulder of the road leading to the elementary school. It was 3.10. When the school bell rung at 3.20, the front of the line would begin to move slowly as one car after another would leave with its child or children. Until then, we mothers and fathers waited. Ahead of me a woman stood by her station wagon watching her preschooler pick up pecans in the grove next to the parked cars. I pulled my car behind hers. She looked familiar. We smiled. She came to the window of my car. 'Hey, how are you?' she asked.

'You mean since my baby died?' The words tumbled out on their own.

'Oh. I'd heard you'd lost a baby,' she said in a voice unnaturally high as if she had just remembered what happened to me. She looked away from me, toward her child.

Suddenly, I felt shunned as if I had a contagious disease. Perhaps she was just making small talk: 'How are you?' could have meant nothing more to her than 'Nice weather we're having.' Then I mentioned my baby dying and we were both without words. I had forgotten how to make small talk. Either I tried to crawl back from being shunned or I tried to assess the meaning of her words when I asked, 'Are you asking to make conversation or do you really want to know how I am since Sarah died?'

'Just making conversation,' she replied crisply as if she wanted this to end quicker than I did.

None of this was her fault. Or mine. The shortest end to the conversation I could think of were two words. 'I'm fine,' I said relieving us both.

Mr Stokes called me a week after Sarah's funeral. 'Theresa, maybe you can help me. Maybe, that is, if you feel like it. It's completely up to you. I just wanted to let you know there is an opening if you are interested. Mrs Burrell, you know Madeline Burrell, the kindergarten aide? Well, her husband is going in for open-heart surgery the first part of next week. If you would like to take over for her for the rest of the year, we'd like to have you back. It will work out to be just about a full month. Do you want to think about it and call me back?'

'I'll be there. What day?'

'Come Monday and meet the children.'

'Thanks.'

Mr Stokes' call was a relief as I didn't want to stay home by myself, and I couldn't always stay at my mother's house. I would be going back to the school routine with friends and coworkers, with children who made me laugh. I knew that grief wouldn't stay at home, but I thought keeping busy in the professional setting would help me have more control over my emotions in the same way that I didn't scream at the funeral as I thought I would. I had never before, in my adult life, had emotions stronger than I was. When I mentioned that to a friend, she commented that for her it was frightening to see another person fall apart. Me, she meant, and just when I felt like, hands down, I was the needy one. Yet, that was part of grief, too, the dealing with friends' emotions over the death of my baby as well as my own emotional reaction. And letting friends know how to help or what helped. It seems like it shouldn't be necessary for the griever to have that responsibility, too, but when none of your friends have buried babies, they don't know what helps and what hurts. Having emotions that intense went against all I'd been taught, beginning with my parents' earliest efforts in socialization, when they admonished me to mind my manners or my temper, to speak pleasantly even to people I did not like and, no, I couldn't ask the lady who lived across the street why she was so fat.

With each first after Sarah my emotions ruled. The first time I drove to the school to teach, I thought about driving to school the last day I'd taught before taking off to have the baby. The remembering contrasted that anticipation with the reality of her short life. Seeing each coworker for the first time, especially the ones I was closest to, would start the tears flowing. I'd duck into bathrooms and sob. But it was just the firsts. When I saw someone or did something for a second time, I could maintain control.

Maybe the way one walks after casts are taken off legs that were broken isn't really walking in any normal sense but moving the legs as if to walk reminds the mind and body how it is done. That's how I felt working as a teacher's aide two weeks after Sarah died. I wasn't really teaching or assisting, even though it might have looked as if I were.

I taught the new kindergarten class a lesson that my own class had enjoyed. Before rain was expected, I read the children a book entitled *Mushrooms in the Rain*. The story tells of the magic and science of mushrooms popping up after the rain. After reading the story, I took the children on a nature walk. We looked for mushrooms, but we didn't see any. The next day – after a rain – we walked the nature trail again. We counted 89 mushrooms and meshed science and magic. Seeing their joy of discovery reminded me of my own joy, weeks earlier, anticipating the new baby's birth when I walked the same nature trail with my own kindergarten class. I walked the last of the nature walk with tears in my eyes and on my cheeks. When the children asked about my tears, I told them that the tears and wet cheeks were from raindrops falling from leaves. They believed me. I couldn't have begun to explain grief to them after we'd counted 89 magic mushrooms.

I learned the children's names. All 27 of them. I didn't think I was capable because, mentally, I wasn't able to think and, physically, I wasn't sleeping or eating much. But I learned their names. In a bizarre, surreal sense, it helped to go through the motions of teaching and of working again even though I felt incapable of either. I thought of the patient in physical therapy who goes through the motions until one day the body can work on its own again. My thoughts were not so lofty; I went through the motions so that I wouldn't be home alone with the pain.

One day I sharpened 27 pencils in preparation for a writing lesson. I shaved points by turning the crank of a mechanical sharpener mounted on the wall. The electric sharpener would not take the fat kindergarten pencils that are about the thickness of three pencils put together. By the time I had sharpened 15, my right thumb ached a bit, but I continued sharpening. During the next three days the joint in my right thumb swelled to nearly twice its normal size, and it hurt. I must have been thinking arthritis because a book entitled *Arthritis* jumped out at me when I was in the library one day with the children. I glanced through the book and six words appeared in large bold type:

Arthritis can harbor group B streptococcus.

I made an appointment with a doctor whose specialty was listed in the phone book as bones and joints. 'Three weeks ago I had a child who died of group B streptococcus. Now I have what I think is arthritis, and I read that arthritis can harbor group B strep. Will I just harbor these bacteria? What if I get pregnant again? Will I lose another baby to group B strep?'

He took my hands into his own and compared the sizes of my thumb joints.

'I'll agree with you about the arthritis. Were you treated after your baby became sick?'

'Yes, with antibiotics.'

'Then that would have killed the strep in your body. You don't have it anymore.'

'But how did I get it? If I got it once and didn't know it, I can get it again, right?'

'Don't worry. Lightning doesn't strike twice in the same place.'

Driving home I was struck by that phrase: 'Lightning doesn't strike twice in the same place.' I heard it over and over. It wouldn't stop playing in my mind until I said out loud. Disease isn't lightning. We can't stop lightning. We can't control the weather, but we can give antibiotics for a strep infection. How unscientific for a doctor to say lightning doesn't strike twice in the same place. What if it were his child? Could he be so sure? Would he be so sure? No, he would read about group B strep and find out how to prevent it from happening to another child of his.

The hospital was not far from our home. I had an hour before Molly would get off the school bus. Emily was at a friend's house until 4.30 p.m. I knew I could do some research in the hospital's library because years ago, I had had a medical question and couldn't find an answer in the local library. A nurse friend suggested I look in the hospital's library.

'Isn't it just for doctors?' I asked.

'Only doctors can check books out of the library, but anybody can go in there and read. Public funds have purchased all the medical books and magazines.'

In the medical center's library, I read the indices of medical journals until I found an article on neonatal group B strep in a journal entitled *OB/GYN*. Doctors in rural hospitals miss the diagnosis for group B strep, it said, more often than doctors in large suburban or urban hospitals. The hospital where Sarah was born was definitely rural. But the doctor who treated Sarah was a neonatologist – a specialist in newborn care as well as illnesses and diseases.

The article continued: 'If antibiotics are administered within the first twelve hours of life, the neonates with group B streptococcus survive.' Sarah was nine hours old when the neonatologist told me that I couldn't have Sarah for the noon feeding, but I could have her at 3.00 p.m. And he was going flying . . . Sarah was born at 2.50 a.m. the day before . . . At 2.00 p.m., after the neonatologist left to go flying, Dr Smith, the doctor on call for him, asked to do chest X-rays because he thought Sarah had pneumonia . . . It was after the X-rays showed that she has pneumonia that she started getting antibiotics . . . It could have been almost 3.00 p.m. before antibiotics were started . . . Sarah didn't get antibiotics until Dr Smith recognized she was sick . . . She was nearly 12 hours old by then.

'In the case of premature rupture of the membranes, the incidence of group B streptococcus is no greater if labor commences within 24 hours.' Amniotic fluid leaked at the sailing club after a late dinner. It must have been 7.30 or 8.00 p.m. Labor started the next night after dinner. We ate dinner at 6.00 p.m. So by 6.30 I was walking. That's when contractions started. Labor started less than 24 hours after amniotic fluid seeped. So I didn't cause Sarah's death by not going to the hospital sooner as the neonatologist had said.

In an article that Carol Baker, MD published two years earlier in *Pediatrics in Review,* she said, 'Full term neonates with no known maternal predisposing factors for infection may develop early onset infection, and those presenting with respiratory distress should be regarded as highly suspect for group B streptococci.' . . . *respiratory distress . . . highly suspect for group B streptococci.* The neonatologist said Sarah had a breathing problem particular to premature infants. I told him Sarah wasn't premature, so he should have suspected something else. But he didn't listen to me. At the time, my joy at Sarah's arrival tempered my anger at the doctor's arrogance because it did not occur to me that she would die – not until she was taken to Wilmington. While reading these articles, I was a mixture of bottomless sadness that her illness was treatable and relief that I had not caused or contributed to her illness and death. Had I believed the 'experts,' the neonatologist and the nurse-midwife, and their mean-spirited remarks that I was selfish and responsible for Sarah's death, I might have remained stuck in grief. To have thought that I caused this nightmare would have been emotionally crippling.

From Dr Baker's article I learned that group B strep is trans-mitted vertically, from mother to baby, and horizontally, from hospital personnel to baby. Babies who become ill before the fifth day of life are said to have an early onset disease, transmitted vertically.

In addition to treating infants with group B strep in the first hours of life, the article said there was a way to prevent the infection from occurring at all: 'The simplicity of obtaining a vaginal culture for streptococcal isolation and the proved vertical transmission of these organisms to neonates with early onset disease are given as reasons to initiate prenatal screening for group B streptococcal colonization.' The bacteria are a 'frequent constituent of the genital bacterial flora in women and men.' My obstetrician could have tested me for strep, treated me with antibiotics, and Sarah would not have gotten sick. Why wasn't I tested?

The article concluded with a statement that should have set off an alarm to all neonatologists, pediatricians, obstetricians, mothers, and fathers: '. . . group B streptococci has been linked to neonatal disease since 1938, but only in the last decade has it become the leading etiologic agent [cause] for bacteremia and/or meningitis occurring during the first two months of life.'

Group B strep is the leading infectious killer of newborns. It is more common than Down Syndrome, spina bifida, and phenylketonuria (PKU) combined, yet for nearly 30 years, parents first heard of the disease when their sick or dead newborns' cultures came back positive for the bacteria.

Dr Baker's interest in group B strep began in 1969, when she was a pediatric resident, and she began seeing infants with an unusual kind of meningitis. In medical school, she'd learned that meningitis contracted in the first month of life is caused by gram-negative bacteria (pink when gram-stained) – but – the babies she was seeing were infected with gram-positive or blue-stained bacteria. The Baylor Affiliated Hospitals laboratory identified the bacteria as a streptococcus but not group B streptococcus because in 1969 it was not believed to be a cause of disease in humans. Within three weeks, this 'new' meningitis took the life of one of Dr Baker's patients, left one with severe brain damage, and another failed to return to normal following severe seizures. Dr Baker asked her senior physicians about this unusual kind of meningitis; the answers did not satisfy her curiosity or her frustration or what became her horror at the death and destruction of beautiful and otherwise healthy newborns.

She began reading old papers dating back as far as 1938 describing GBS infections in a handful of pregnant women and newborns. She also studied the recent cases at the Baylor hospitals and found patterns in the onset of the disease, the symptoms and signs, and the outcomes.

'I had the brilliant (in retrospect) foresight to save the bacteria isolated from these cases. Seeing as I knew little about microbiology, only the hardy nature of GBS allowed their survival,' she told me. She sent these bacteria to Dr Rebecca Lancefield at the Rockefeller University in New York whose classification system for streptococcus is still used today. Dr Lancefield was excited about Dr Baker's streptococcus because the overwhelming majority was a type that she had only uncommonly encountered since she developed her system in the 1930s. Later Dr Lancefield invited Dr Baker to study with her in New York where she learned the typing and beginnings of the chemistry of the organization.

Dr Baker's article was rejected by the first journal she sent it to with the comment that group B strep was 'nothing more than a localized phenomena in Texas.' The year her article was published, 1979, the bacterium was the leading cause of death of newborns by infectious disease and remained so for nearly two more decades, after approximately 400 000 babies in the US alone died or suffered from its devastating physical and mental disorders.

12. Hove to

A storm at sea can be avoided by going ashore or sailing into a cove where the violent winds are choked off by land and trees. Sometimes, though, the shore is too far away or no coves are nearby, and the storm cannot be dodged. Strong winds can capsize a boat or rip the sails and snap the stays, the metal ropes that support the mast, or crack the rudder or centerboard. Each tear, each broken stay, each splintered piece of wood, each crack in the fiberglass makes the boat more susceptible to further damage. When sailing in rough weather is not an option, a safe way to weather the storm is to adjust the sails a certain way called hove to. Hove to stops forward motion, allowing the boat to ride out the storm at sea.

Before I was pregnant with Sarah, Tom and I were caught in one of those summer storms that built so quickly that outrunning it to a cove or shoreline was impossible and sailing through it was too risky for our little boat. We had only read about hove to; we'd never tried it in good weather or in bad. The storm was battering us with strong winds and rain; the sails protested by alternately filling and slapping against the stays, spilling their air as high waves rocked the boat. Proceeding on course was becoming dangerous. We came into the wind, that is we steered the boat directly into the wind so that the bow was facing the wind and the main and jib sails flapped like flags. We tied the main sail down tightly by pulling in the mainsheet as far as the rope would allow, close hauled it's called. Then, still into the wind, we tied down the jibsheet tightly, too, but the jib was on the other side of the boom. The bird's-eye view of sails in hove to is a dollar sign with a single line drawn through the middle. We drifted downwind, creating a slick in the choppy water. The slick, a protective slick it's called, blunted the force of the waves as they broke well to our windward, before they reached us, and long before they could toss the boat. A sailboat is built to sail, so it naturally tries to sail even when hove to. We dragged an anchor at the bow, as we drifted backward, thus keeping the boat from creeping forward and attempting to sail. If we had to ride out the storm, hove to was a safe way to do so. We didn't make any progress, but our boat wasn't battered and broken by waves and wind too strong for our little craft.

There's a time, too, while grieving to hove to. Weeks after Sarah, the shock of her death began to become a reality and the longest and loneliest stage of grieving began. I was like a dog licking my wounds; I found corners in rooms or in my mind for myself and my sorrow. The forays I made into the world were physical only; mentally I lived in a cocoon that only began to unravel months later. Grieving is typically a year-long process that is particularly sad during the first six months; after that the heaviest weight lifts. But when death comes without warning, when it is as unexpected and tragic as death from a car accident, or suicide, or murder, or after a problem-free pregnancy, grieving is longer than a year. Three years in these cases is more the norm; some experts say two to four years is to be expected after the death of a child. Grief mirrors love: its depths are in proportion to its heights – its breadth in proportion to the loss. The death of an aged grandmother who's lived a life of fulfilled dreams is a loss surely, a loss of what was, but the death of a baby that one planned to share life with, is a loss of what was to be, what should have been. One is the loss of your past; the other is the loss of your future.

My cousin Ann called from her home in West Virginia, 'Where are you in the stages of grieving?' she asked.

'I've been through them all,' I told her. 'I've been through shock, denial, anger, depression. Well, all but acceptance.'

In reality, the stages of grief that I'd experienced in those early weeks were more like fireworks; I'd had flashes of denial, anger, and depression, but I was too steeped in shock to experience them fully, to deal with them completely. In the weeks after Sarah, as I could take in the meaning of her death, I became aware of how much I had lost.

Grief had a bottomless black hole. At first, the sides sloped gently then they became tiered ledges, and the grade increased dramatically. The fear of slipping in was more frightening than any fear I had ever known. Somehow I knew that if I fell into the black hole, I would struggle forever and without success to get out. The danger of slipping was always present but at times was more imminent. It was worse when I accidentally found the baby blanket that I made for Sarah, the yellow-checked one edged in eyelet lace. Hot tears spilled over my cheeks, debilitating me, and I stumbled from flat ground to a tiered ledge overlooking the black hole. I wondered what I ever did to deserve Sarah's death. And I stumbled again, closer. I was not strong enough to resist the pull. I felt my father's large hand squeezing my little one. We were on our first 'date,' the father-daughter night at the National Press Club in Washington, D.C. I was seven years old, and my new patent leather pumps pinched my toes. My heels are so narrow that I select shoes too short for my feet so I won't walk out of them. My father's squeezes made my shoes not hurt; they made all things right. I wished for another squeeze . . . my brother Joe whistles; Little Joe smiles . . . the scenes marched through my mind like band members in a parade, relentless, and I slipped further toward the black hole. The only way to keep from slipping all the way into the blackness was to stop the parade. I would begin doing something, anything, with a frenzy: rake leaves, vacuum, walk the hall, phone Kath or my mother, or give Daisy a dog biscuit. I did not fall into the blackness that time. The effort to keep from falling would leave me breathless. My heart would race.

As I would drive the curvy blacktop road to my mother's house, I would see Sarah's face in a mirage on the road. Her eyelashes would be brushing her round, full cheeks. I would speed up to get a closer look, but the image would disappear with the mirage.

And I would be stung by grief for the thousandth time that day, no, that hour.

I wanted to shed the grief, but not the look, smell, feel or sound of Sarah. I would hold her in my mind and in my dreams. I would wake from snatches of sleep to realize that the dream of her nuzzling between my arm and my body was only a dream. Waking was horror. I couldn't stop what was happening to me. I could only control a small part of my reaction to it. I stopped sleeping real sleep. I applauded myself for sleeping lightly. Mornings were easier that way. I was getting better I thought – mornings without horror. Better? My God, what an existence – avoiding horror.

I became a walking zombie from lack of sleep. I would walk into a room and wouldn't know why I had gone there. Sometimes I would open my mouth to speak and wouldn't know what I had intended to say or, other times, words that barely began to express a thought would hang, suspended, and neither I nor the person I was talking with could do anything to complete the unfinished remark. I asked my neighbor of two years what his name was. I watched people look at me, a zombie, and I wondered if there was any difference between grief and insanity.

Mostly, those forays into the world were like dodging into and out of a battleground, and I felt way under armed. I went to the grocery store for bread, milk, taco shells, and hot dogs. I collected everything except the bread. When I turned the grocery cart into the aisle where the bread was shelved, I saw a kelly-green infant seat cradling a newborn. The seat rested in the mother's grocery cart. To pick out a loaf of bread, I would have to push my cart past the baby in the infant seat. I decided that we did not need bread that week; we would do without.

On a Sunday, I went downtown to the Central News and Card Shop. I selected several more boxes of stationery for what had become my ongoing occupation – writing thank you notes for food and flowers and money that kept arriving. The woman behind the counter recognized me. Her grin was wide and happy. 'You had the baby, I see. What did you have?'

'A girl. But she died.' She apologized for not knowing, for bringing up the subject. I told her, please, not to be sorry. I was grateful that she had acknowledged what many people avoided mentioning.

Leslie Plaster shopped at Big Star where I bought most of my groceries. We were acquainted because our husbands were foresters who worked at Weyerhaeuser. Leslie and Alan sent a hanging plant after Sarah died. The tiny heart-shaped leaves cascaded from the basket in thick emerald green clusters. The plant is appropriately named baby tears. I saw Leslie at the meat counter as we sorted through packages of ground beef. When she asked how I was, I wondered if she really wanted to know.

'I haven't seen you since the funeral,' she added. Her eyes met mine. They did not seem afraid of someone else's pain. They did not look away; they searched for answers or a communion of souls.

I told her about my dreams of holding Sarah in my arms and of waking up. She did not look away. I told her that missing Sarah was not just in the morning; it was all the time. She did not look away. She listened to my description of sorrow. She listened without judging me or my emotions. She didn't try to fix me, as others had, or tell me that it couldn't be *that* bad, or tell me that Sarah's death was God's will or in God's plan or that He needed another angel in heaven or that I could have another baby – none of which helped. She just listened, affirming me and the journey I was on. I thanked her for the visit, picked up my package of ground beef, and knew I would carry that moment forever.

Alone or in a crowd, I would feel something on the back of my hand or on my arm or just above my knee. I would look to see my own fingertips moving ever so gently. The touch was light, much as I'd use to stroke the feverish forehead of a sick child. When I first noticed my fingers brushing my skin, I thought I must have been trying to soothe myself.

Molly and Emily would play too quietly in the playroom in those early weeks after Sarah. They were too good. I was relieved they did not need me because I was too busy avoiding the black hole to tend to them much.

I nicked a fingernail and the ragged edge threatened to snag a stocking or worse begin a rip that would take the whole nail off at the quick. I dug through my purse until I found a nail file, settled into the comfy chair in the living room, and began to smooth the ragged edge with the fine steel file when my eyes started to burn. A couple of weeks earlier, I'd filed my nails and Sarah was making little bulges pop up on my stomach, hard little knots made with her feet or elbows or knees. Tom and I lay in bed that night and watched the movements and imagined the shape of the baby's body. Tom put an ice cube on my stomach, and we laughed as the baby squirmed to find a warmer spot. If I filed my nails again, I would sever another connection to Sarah; I stopped filing.

My mother asked, 'If I were to take you out to dinner, what would you like to eat?'

'I'm not really hungry, Mom, but thanks.'

'Honey, I know you're not hungry. But if you were, what would you like to eat?'

'Flounder. Do you remember when I was pregnant, I couldn't get enough fish?' Normally I don't eat much fish – just during Lent. Although I hadn't attended Mass on Sundays in years, I still abstained from eating meat on Fridays during Lent out of habit. Fresh flounder here on the coast is the best. Yes, flounder, if I were hungry.

'Tonight, let me pick you up – you and Tom and Molly and Emily,' my mother told me. 'I'll take you all to dinner. I'll pick you up at 5.30.'

We went to a favorite fish house, the one we go to to take some-one out for a birthday dinner, the one with white cloth tablecloths and napkins, the one with fresh flowers on the tables and candles and soft music. My plate was full of fillet of flounder, a baked potato yellow with butter, and fashionably long green beans adorned with slivered almonds. Paprika was sprinkled over the feather-like folds of the flounder's white meat.

'If I felt like getting better, I would eat,' I told my mother.

'Pick up your fork,' she said, not as a mother would to a young child, but in a coaxing, firm manner – not a matter for discussion. I picked up my fork and ate what tasted like cotton.

Grief, like the humidity of August in the deep south, permeated all my pores, it invaded my mind and my emotions, diminishing my joys and intensifying my fears. Like the waves at high tide that cover the hot sandy beaches as they stretch toward castles of sand to break them down, grief pounds incessantly, wallowing out my spirit, my sense of optimism and my hope.

I was hove to as the storm raged on. Yes, I was battered by grief, but what I didn't know at the time was that I was doing more than reacting to the storm – I was working, doing some of the hardest work I'd ever done. Part of the job of grieving is to make sense of the senseless, to find a reason to go on, to answer questions like: Why am I here? What's important? What do I want? Before I die, what do I want to have accomplished? Grief tore me apart, and as I put the pieces of me back together in a new and redirected order, I was more firm on some issues, more open on others, less judgmental. My fears were different. I found extraordinary in the ordinary and gratitude for all I had, my family, my children, Tom. These would be years in the coming.

13. A solitary journey

Most bereaved parents suffer from marital difficulty within months after the death of their child.

The Bereaved Parent

Tom's boss, Thurston, called me June 6, one month to the day after Sarah was buried, the day the hourly workers refused to sign their contract.

'T, how are you holding up?'

'Thurston, there are days I think I'm going to make it, and there are days when I don't think I can bear the pain.'

'Sweetheart, you're in our prayers. We're looking after Tom here at work and thinking of you. Look, something's come up. I'm asking you first. If you say, no, that's it. I won't ask Tom. And there won't be any problem – either way. Understand?'

'I can say yes or no. But what am I saying yes or no to?'

'You've heard about the possible strike at the mill?' Thurston asked.

'Sure, Tom took the bus-driving course in case we had a strike.'

'Well, we do. Salaried workers, for now, are taking over the jobs at the mill. We need Tom to do his job and, if you okay it, to drive a bus and work at the mill some, too. Can you manage evenings and weekends by yourself?'

'How long do you think this strike will last?'

'It's anybody's guess.'

'Tom wouldn't feel right not doing his part if everyone else is working extra hours. Sure, Thurston.' Tom and I had known the hourly workers might strike; we'd known long before Sarah's birth and death. We knew, also, since Sarah, that it would be difficult for both of us if he worked so many hours. The up side was, Tom would be paid overtime.

The strike at the Weyerhaeuser Company polarized our town and changed the course of Tom's and my grief. The hourly workers refused to sign the annual contract and walked off their jobs at the paper mill in protest. The contract had two fewer paid holidays and a decrease in medical benefits – the equivalent of a $400 pay cut or an average of two weeks' pay. The decrease in medical benefits came as the cost of medical care began to shoot up 27% in one year.

I dreaded the first morning Tom left to work the strike. We got up at 5.15. I fixed breakfast and made sandwiches, put cookies in a baggie, and washed an apple for his lunch. Already it was 5.45 and he was kissing me goodbye. Then he was gone, and I was alone until Molly and Emily woke up.

After Sarah died and before the strike began, I had followed Tom everywhere. I followed him to the bathroom and watched him shave. If he made a phone call, I was in the same room. If he changed the oil in his truck, I opened up a lawn chair and set it beside the truck. I would sit there until he tossed all the empty oil cans into the garbage can and covered the drips of oil with kitty litter. If he bought gas, I gathered Molly and Emily and rode to the station with him. When he had a root canal filled at the dentist's office a ten-minute drive from our house, I sat in the dentist's waiting room. For that first month when Tom was home I was by his side. When I'd told my mother that I'd follow him around, she asked how that made Tom feel. I wasn't thinking much about his feelings, but I did then and told her that Tom was basking in his new role. 'Do you want something?' he'd asked me at first when I'd follow him to the bedroom as he changed from work clothes to a T-shirt and shorts. 'No,' I'd tell him. 'I just want to be near you.' Then his questions changed. 'I'm just going to my truck to get my briefcase. Want to come along?' he'd ask, giving me a second to put down my book or sewing before we'd leave the room. And so it was for the month after Sarah until I told Thurston yes.

How could I have told Thurston yes, I wondered that first morning of the strike? What was I thinking? I was not ready to be without him in the mornings before Molly and Emily woke. My fear frightened me. I was out of breath. I couldn't scream or the girls would hear me. I couldn't sleep. I couldn't sit or read or watch TV. So, I did something I have never done before or since. Just after Tom left, at 5.45, while it was still dark outside, while Molly and Emily slept, I ran. I ran the route the school bus takes to get to our house; I ran to the highway and back toward home.

I ran from our house to the edge of the black neighborhood and back again. I ran for miles. A man on a bicycle rode toward me. I couldn't tell who he was or what he was wearing; it was too dark. As I passed him, I glanced his way ever so quickly. I had never seen him before. He stopped his bicycle, put his feet on the pavement and looked at me as if to speak. I stared at him and for the first time in my life, I was not afraid of coming so close to a man of another race on the street whom I didn't know when I was by myself, in the dark, and not near home. I had other fears now. I passed him and heard the crunching of his rubber tires as they rolled over the sand and worn pebbles that poked above the asphalt. The sounds became fainter. Finally I ran home and stopped moving. Every muscle started to shake. I had energy only to weep; I could not scream.

When Molly and Emily woke, I went through the motions of the normal summer-day routine: serve breakfast, wash dishes, get the girls to take their dirty clothes to the laundry room, wash clothes, coordinate play time with friends, watch cartoons, shop for groceries, make lunch, read the comics, read stories before naps, take them to the swimming pool, make dinner. I cared for them but connected with them only on a superficial level. It was a hollow kind of caring but all I was capable of doing. Emily told me she wanted her mommy to be mommy again.

'Is Sarah scared of the dark?' Emily asked.

'It's not dark in heaven so Sarah doesn't have any dark to be scared of. She's in a happy place.'

'But she doesn't have her mommy.'

'Well, no. But she has angels to play with and Jesus. And in heaven you're not lonely.'

'Why did she die?'

'She got sick.'

'Don't cry, Mommy. Swing me.' Emily loved the swing in the backyard. Hung from a branch high in a massive oak tree, the swing carried her nearly to Mrs Rhodes' yard before it would stall for a delicious moment in space and time as it gathered momentum to make its way back for another, 'Push, Mommy.' I pushed the swing an average of 20 times a day as I had since we moved to this house when she was eight months old.

'Push me higher.'

I hadn't pushed Emily on the swing since Sarah. Maybe she hadn't asked me. Maybe I hadn't heard her ask. It was another first. Emily giggled and screamed with pleasure.

'Higher,' she yelled.

I pushed harder.

She made a sound that scared me – as if she had been stung by a bee. I caught her legs as they swooshed at me. 'Emily, honey, what's the matter?'

'I wanted Sarah,' she sobbed.

We hugged. She in the swing, me kneeled below. 'Me, too,' I told her. Grief ambushes children in mid-swing, and sometimes when they are doing the thing they love most. They don't grieve as adults do. They play and cry when ambushed.

Molly and Em and I had been connected by jokes, by needing hugs, by curling our hair together, by peanut-butter-sandwich lunches in the park, by decorating sugar cookies with colored frosting and sprinkles, by learning how to pucker up and whistle, by 'winking' – holding our eye-lids closed with our fingers, by holding hands and skipping, by reading some poems so many times that we memorized them. By Molly and I singing off-key, Emily on-key, and Tom mocking us by howling like a dog whose ears hurt. We had been connected by homemade Halloween costumes: Molly the bride, Emily the bridesmaid.

'If you'll empty the trash, I'll fix your hair.'

'If you'll drive me to Allison's house, I'll read to Emily before she takes a nap.'

We were also connected by shopping trips for baby toys, by deciding where to hang the mobile over the crib, by washing miniature undershirts and gowns and folding them together and stacking them on the baby's changing table. But grief robbed us of us.

'Hold me, Mom,' Molly said one day. 'Here, in this rocking chair. Hold me. My stomach hurts.'

I held her and pushed on the balls of my feet until the rocker drifted backward; I stopped pushing and the rocker tipped forward. Molly held her Acey and stared at nothing. Before Sarah, I would have kissed her hair and asked her what she was thinking. I would have squeezed her until she giggled. I would have slipped one of my fingers inside her tiny fist to feel its warmth, its softness, its squeeze. But I stared at nothing that summer and so did she. We were two people who happened to be in the same rocking chair.

Molly said, 'Mom, my stomach doesn't hurt when you hold me.'

I rested my chin lightly on the blonde curls on top of her head and closed my eyes to keep them from stinging.

Nothing about that summer was normal. I lived on edge. I startled easily. If a door slammed unexpectedly, I shuddered. If one of the girls called for me in that I-need-you-right-now tone of voice, my fight or flight adrenalin kicked in as I imagined one of them either badly injured or in danger. They weren't. Maybe a shoelace had come untied. For the months the strike continued, for the months I lived without Tom's companionship, I ran in a panic when they called me. When the phone rang, I trembled, afraid of bad news.

After dinner, without Tom, the girls and I mowed the grass, replaced the screen wire in doors and windows, raked the lawn of pecan shells, potted plants, trimmed bushes, walked, rode bikes, went to the park to swing, to pass the time until midnight when Tom would come home. The neighbors commented that the yard had never looked so neat. I didn't tell them that I had to keep busy. Grieving without Tom was like treading water. If I stopped moving I would go under. I didn't know what the 'under' was but I knew it was there and it was black and deep. It frightened me into frenzied, water treading activity. Maybe if I stopped, I would cry. Not the crying I did every morning on waking and realizing I had to again face the day without Sarah, or the tears that came when I balanced the checkbook and saw the check I'd written to the neonatologist for Sarah. I wasn't afraid anymore of the regular tears. But I was afraid of not moving, that I might start crying, sobbing, screaming and never stop. If I stopped moving, I might never move again. If I stopped moving, I thought about life without Sarah.

At night after the girls went to sleep, I'd read books about the grief process from parents' points of view and psychiatrists', therapists', and counselors'. *Motherhood and Mourning,* a book about perinatal death, reaffirmed my experience in the lack of community support after a baby dies, saying that the baby had not become part of the community. In interviews with mothers of babies who had died, they spoke of hospital staff members and physicians who discarded the intense emotions of shock and grief with statements like, 'Perk up. You can have another baby.' *When Pregnancy Fails* said the grief process could take from 6 to 24 months. Those books validated my experiences with hospital personnel who were acting on the best medical knowledge at the time: that stillborn, newborn, and infant death would not generate reactions of grief. It wouldn't be until the 1990s that the medical profession would begin to realize that the death of a child at any age was a sad event for the mother and the family. In the book *When a Baby Dies* published in 1990, the author, Irving G Leon says,

> Until about ten years ago, the medical profession had demonstrated a startling lack of sensitivity and responsiveness to the often traumatizing impact of perinatal loss. Physicians typically denied or minimized the significance of the loss, avoided discussing the death with parents, prescribed sedatives to reduce expressions of maternal shock and grief, discouraged or prohibited contact with the dead baby, and recommended having another child as soon as possible rather than recognize the necessity of grieving in resolving the death (48).

It would be even years later that the medical community would discover that the death of a child, whether a newborn or an adult, was the worst loss. In 1994, Barbara D Rosof published *The Worst Loss* saying, 'A stillbirth or the death of a newborn is as great a loss as the death of a young adult (14). Even before a child is conceived, parents have fantasized about it, endowed it with their hopes and longings (9)'. The author/psychotherapist says losing a child is the worst loss because the damage to families' lives is much broader than that of any other loss. Husbands and wives have a difficult time communicating because never before had they both been so needy at the same time. (That wasn't Tom's and my problem during the strike; he wasn't home enough for us to try to communicate.) Children are the forgotten mourners.

Books available about the death of newborns in 1981 did not begin to touch on the extreme emotions I was experiencing. When I began reading books about deaths of older children, I felt connected to other people who had felt what I was feeling. I learned tips to functioning during those early months of grief. Harriet Sarnoff Schiff writing in *The Bereaved Parent* says cry no more than ten minutes at a time. I was not responsible for the emotions that brought on the tears, but I was responsible for how long I let them flow. 'When the mind is tired, exercise the body. When the body is tired, exercise the mind,' one of the books admonished. So, when I raised blisters from raking pecan shells, I'd sit and read. When printed words blurred and my eyes stung, I'd talk Molly and Em into walking around the block with me or going to the park to seesaw or slide. The sudden shift from mind to body or body to mind had a healing effect because I was in control of part of my life. *Most marriages do not survive the death of a child,* I read. So take care of your marriage, the author continued, because you have already lost enough. And: unless suicide is an option the only way to the other side of grief is through it. I read, too, that some people never get to the other side. Although some of my relatives had taken their own lives, it was not something I considered. I also learned that by doing what I was doing, caring for the girls as best I could, doing laundry, shopping for groceries, cooking, all while feeling the loss, that I was doing the necessary work of grieving, and I would get better, the pain would lessen and I would find joy in life again. I learned there was a vast difference between what people expected of me and what I could expect from myself. I learned that people who have never buried a loved one might think grieving is over when the funeral is over and the person goes back to work, or school, or buys groceries. My reactions were normal; I was not going insane. Printed words assured me I would be able to function again, but I would always miss Sarah.

An entry in Tom's diary says that June 16 through 18 my mother, Carl and I took the girls to Williamsburg, Virginia to see Pete, who was working at Busch Gardens as a guitar player. The girls wore the T-shirts their uncle had given them with the words: *Pete's my uncle* in four-inch-high metallic letters.

The weekend of June 20 was Tom's first weekend home in 18, his diary says, as either fire duty or strike duty had kept him working. The following weekend, he was off, too, and we went sailing with the Sellers. Just as Tom was sailing out of our sailing club's cove, he tacked, and Molly fell, hitting her head against the metal teeth of the centerboard wench. The wound required seven stitches and left a scar through what would otherwise have been a widow's peak hairline. The Sellers waited for us to get back from the emergency room before we sailed side-by-side for our two-day trip to Beard Creek. Their three-week-old son, Chris, stayed with his grandparents. For dinner that night, Molly, Em, and Jennifer roasted hot dogs and marshmallows on the beach. Even with Molly's head wrapped in enough adhesive tape so that she appeared to be wearing a helmet, it was a good weekend, a time to be with Barbara and Preston again and watch our girls play and hear them laugh. Barbara and Preston were gentle with our emotions, somehow understanding that we were walking wounded. They didn't ask that we snap out of it or get back to normal or be brave for the children. They just accepted us where we were.

Vera was upset when she invited Emily and me for a visit that summer, but she graciously made small talk for a while. Molly must have been at a friend's house that day or visiting Grammie.

'How about a cup of coffee?' she asked tilting in her white wicker porch chair. The uneven brick floor was laid that way intentionally to appear antebellum. Screened on three sides, the porch provided a wide view of the Trent River, of recreational boats, of fishermen, of birds, of fish jumping and shining in the sun. The sight of the river was through ragged sheets of Spanish moss draped over branches of loblolly pine trees. Sunlight danced off the waves.

'No, thanks.'

'Whatsamadda? Are you sick or somethin?' my friend asked.

'I don't drink coffee anymore.'

'You are sick.'

'No, I just don't need any more stimulation. I feel too much already.'

She brought me a cup of decaffeinated coffee and we talked about our girls, Emily and Jena, who are the same age and about her husband Steve's sailboat that had just sunk in the front 'yard'. His boat is the same as ours – a San Juan 21.

'Tell me about the shed,' I said finally, the source of her angst. She stood up and asked me to follow her. Next to her house away from the view from the porch was the new aluminum shed, the one my brother Carl and his girlfriend, Cara, had assembled. Vera showed me how the doors wouldn't close properly. I wished Carl and Cara had taken the doors off and put them back on correctly. I didn't want this to come between us.

'What makes me mad is the olives,' she said.

'Olives?'

'Carl said he would put this together for $40 and two chef's salads with olives. We were out of olives so I drove all the way into town that morning for olives. And now look at this door. Cara said they were not coming back to fix it.'

'I'm sorry you made a special trip. He was only playing with you about the olives.' I thought about offering to fix it myself, but that's not the problem – making a nice salad and getting shoddy work was.

'Don't worry about it,' she said, but I knew she was hurt. We walked back to the porch. Once seated she asked, 'So, your water broke?'

'It seeped a little. It wasn't continuous. Just sometimes when I walked. Not when I was standing or sitting or lying down.'

'But you didn't go to the hospital right away?'

'I called the doctor right away, but he wasn't concerned. Later he said that there would be a risk of infection if contractions didn't start for 24 hours, but they started before 24 hours.'

I felt interrogated. Guilty. Yet, Vera would not interrogate me. Vera's husband is a pediatrician. Are doctors in our town discussing Sarah's illness? Do they blame me, too? What does Vera know? Whose side is she on? Why do I feel as if there are sides? Before Sarah, Vera and I were together. Is my guilt making me feel as if there is a gulf between us? The temperature was in the 80s, yet I was cold and wished I were home. Forays back into the world were difficult. I wasn't initiating visits with friends, so I was grateful that Vera had reached out to me.

Tom's diary says that my mother and my brothers were frequent visitors that summer, and that we often went to dinner at their house. The Sellers and the Manzenes took us out to dinner many times that summer, Tom's diary says, and that Kath and Glenda took me on shopping trips, yet I have no memory of those dinners or shopping trips.

As the summer and the strike progressed, the hours Tom and the other managers were working began to take their toll. One marriage ended. The manager came home to see two tracks in his front yard left by a moving truck. His wife had left and taken all the furniture. The strike workers only came home to sleep and change clothes, and in the beginning – to eat dinner. Like Tom, they were only sleeping five hours a night. Wives of other managers told stories of their husbands falling asleep in the shower or during sex. Once Tom fell asleep while eating dinner: his head dropped into his bowl of soup bumping his nose and causing a bruise. Startled, he woke up. Molly, Emily, and I helped him walk to bed. Tom told me he slept at red lights until the blasts of horns by annoyed motorists would wake him. Months or years later, when there was time to reflect, Tom told me that his experience working two jobs mirrored mine at home. We both kept busy constantly that first summer to cope with and work through a lot of our grief.

I was pregnant that first summer after Sarah, but only for a few weeks, and as with the other early miscarriages, it ended in a spontaneous abortion that did not require a doctor or hospital visit. For those pregnant weeks, I was lifted out of grief and into hope. After years of infertility, I was elated that I could get pregnant. The miscarriage was sad, yes, but the early miscarriages did not involve the huge hormone shift that later ones do. I think even while trying to conceive that summer, part of me knew that, not pregnant, I would devote more time to doing the work of grieving and be better able, later, to welcome a new baby and nurture my family again.

Since there wasn't a sound from the girls, I assumed they were asleep. I laid in bed that summer morning wishing I could avoid the day when Molly was silently and suddenly standing by my side. She had flour on her nose and in her hair. She was holding a wooden spoon that dripped batter onto my bedspread.

'When you're making waffles, what does it mean to fold the batter?' she asked.

I imagined the kitchen dusted with flour, pots and pans pulled out of cupboards, eggs rolling around the counter top skirting the edge, drops of warm margarine oozing from the corners of the folded waxed paper covering, the dog licking sugar granules off the floor below the counter top where a measuring cup had turned over, spilled milk running under the plugged-in toaster. I left my bed like a rocket launching. In the kitchen, I saw that my imagination had not let me down. The dog was not eating sugar granules but was licking ice cream from its cardboard container.

'I gave Daisy some ice cream so she wouldn't wake you, Mom,' Emily said.

I didn't yell or scream. But I made them clean up, and I reminded them that they were not to cook without me even if they were trying to surprise me. It was then that I promised myself to take my mother up on her offer to take me shopping for a new dress.

'What may I help you with?' The tall, slender, black-haired shop owner asked as I rifled through a rack of expensive dresses in the shop owned by my mother's neighbor. I didn't tell her that I would like a new dress to reward myself for getting out of bed when I wanted to take the phone off the hook, lock the doors, pull the covers over my head, and make mental lists of all the reasons I had to feel sorry for myself. I didn't tell her that I decided to buy myself a new dress after Molly and Emily tried to make waffles by themselves.

'I'd like something sexy. I've lost a little weight and I want to show off.' My mother's purchase was an emerald green sundress with a fitted bodice and a full gored skirt in a size eight.

In July, the weekend of the Dog Days Regatta, a sailboat race, Tom got a substitute for his strike job, and we entered our first race since Sarah. The race is named after the wind in July, which is normally light to nonexistent. As it turned out, the wind was unusually brisk, even gusty at times. The well-marked course was laid out on a wide part of the Neuse River flanked by high orange bluffs.

Tom said he thought we could win the race, as many regular winners were not competing. We set our sails and beat to windward toward the first marker with the other boats, testing the wind before the starting gun sounded. We looked like water beetles as we zig-zagged in and out of each other's paths. The wind freshened, picked up a bit, and I had trouble catching my breath. The gun went off and all the boats sailed quickly across the starting line almost in a queue. I had more trouble trying to breathe.

Before Sarah, the excitement of the competition – the shoutings of the captains and crews, the loud flappings of sails of tacking boats, the sights of the other boats and crew so close I could touch the competition – all worked to exhilarate me. 'Pull in the mainsheet,' I'd yell to Tom or I'd reach over and pull the boom toward me until he could adjust the mainsheet. That was before Sarah. Now I couldn't breathe. 'Let the sail out!' I shouted.

'But we'll lose.' He looked at me incredulously, ripped off his hat, threw it in the wet bottom of the boat, sending water splashing, and shouted, 'Damn!'

My chest compressed as I worked harder to inhale. I took big gulps of air, but my lungs would not accept them. My fingers tingled, my toes were numb, and white pinpoints of light jumped at me. Tom spilled the air, the boat slowed and with it my anxiety did, too.

Tom leaned forward in his seat on the deck watching the boats ahead of us get smaller. He squinted his eyes and creases formed in the corners, yet there was no glaring sun – it was more like he was in pain. The boats were passing us by, but life itself was passing us by. I would heal and again become a competitive racer, but ten weeks after Sarah, competition was more fearful than challenging.

In our Christmas letter of 1981, Tom would call the year one of tragedy and triumph. The triumph was a house. In July, Woody, our friend from the sailing club, called to say that he had accepted a job out of state and if we still wanted to buy his and Carol's house, he wouldn't advertise it. Four years earlier, Woody and

Carol had invited us to dinner. When we drove into their driveway for the first time, Tom and I elbowed each other at once; we were in awe of the wood-sided house on a lot with many trees, and a garden spot, a playhouse, and a swing. So in one breath we said hi to our friends and asked them to call us if they ever wanted to sell their house. Woody laughed and said that he'd heard that before, and yes, it was likely that they'd move, though he didn't know when. That summer after Sarah, I handled the paper work for buying the home and made preparations, like hiring a painter, to put ours on the market. I remember being pleased about the move but not elated as I would have been before Sarah. In contrast, I was not worried about owning two homes and two mortgages as Woody and Carol would not sell their home contingent upon the sale of our home, and that year, interest rates skyrocketed to 22%. Before Sarah, I would have worried about the loans and the gamble we were taking, but when my worst fears became reality, all other problems paled in significance.

In July, we rented a vacation home on the Neuse River for a week, one that belonged to a teacher-friend of mine. Tom's boss, Thurston, did not hesitate to give Tom the time off from working the strike and his regular job. Vacations were not the norm that summer of the strike, but Thurston must have been thinking of Sarah when he told Tom yes. Tom's parents, brothers and their families joined us. What stands out for me that week was hearing my brother Pete play a gig at a club nearby. While there, I saw a woman I knew from the sailing club who worked as a counselor at the local mental health center. She asked me how I was doing, and I told her I didn't think I was doing very well because, unlike Tom, I had to talk about Sarah all the time. I still felt so needy; I couldn't sleep unless I was curled up next to Tom spoon-like. I told her about the sailboat race and the anxiety attack. She reminded me that as the mother, I had bonded with Sarah more than Tom. It was okay, she said, to be needy and to grieve differently. Maybe Tom's appearance of strength, she continued, is his desire to be there for you. This may be one of the first times in your married lives that he has been in a position to help you. Let him. You'll be able to do something for him someday, she said. Her words were gifts that freed me to do what I was doing, without guilt, and to not push myself to grieve faster; grief has its own timetable. She said, also, that she didn't think we were meant to get by without other people, that grief puts us in touch with our humanity. I asked her how she could counsel people who had buried a child if she had not had that experience. She said grief is the same whether your friend moves away or your spouse dies. You are surprised or shocked, you deny that the event took place, you get depressed and angry and finally you accept. The only difference between your friend moving away and your spouse dying is the intensity. In that one word, *intensity*, lies all the difference, I thought.

As the strike continued from weeks into months, the corporate executives knew that working such hours was stressful. To compensate, chefs were flown in from Tacoma, Washington, the corporate home office, to cook for the replacement mill workers. Alaskan king crab legs, fresh seafood gumbo, orange roughy, shrimp scampi, lobster, chateaubriand, T-bone steaks, and prime rib roast were served for lunches and dinners. Platters of eggs, mounds of thick, sliced, slab bacon and Canadian bacon, rib eye steaks, homemade pastries, biscuits, fluffy pancakes with Vermont maple syrup, and fresh fruit platters were served for breakfasts. Foods that were not available locally were flown in. Flights bringing fresh seafood or seasoned meats arrived two or three times a week. Tom and the other replacement workers stopped eating meals at home. They all gained weight.

Managers working double shifts or two jobs brought home paychecks two or three times their normal salary while their family lives were nonexistent and adequate sleep was a memory. The striking hourly workers sold their motor homes or fishing boats, took out second mortgages, worked pumping gas or bagging groceries to hold out and hold on until the end of the strike. Months went by and neither side was winning. The strike seemed to be about power rather than a cut in pay.

In early August, two months after the strike began, a woman from the neonatologist's office called.

'The autopsy results are in.'

'Fine, just send them to me.'

'You wouldn't be able to understand them. The doctor will explain them to you. He can see you at 2.30 p.m. on Tuesday the 18th, that's the third Tuesday of next month. I'll put you down for that time.'

'My husband would like to hear the results too. I can't make an appointment without checking with him to see if that's convenient.'

'Call and we'll try to work you in.'

Hearing the results and seeing the neonatologist again were two things that I could not do without Tom. The neonatologist had told me not to have an autopsy performed. Could the autopsy show something he didn't want me to know? Could it show who was at fault? Since we paid for the autopsy, why were the results sent to him? Could he change the results? Would he select information to give me and information to withhold? Would the autopsy report remain in his possession? Why couldn't I have it? I didn't know how Tom could make time to go with me to the neonatologist's office.

For weeks the note about making an appointment with the neonatologist stayed in a pile of things for Tom. The pile included a letter from his mother, a flyer about an upcoming foresters' conference to be held at his alma mater, Virginia Polytechnic Institute, information about a photography contest that he'd requested, a letter from his childhood friend Gordon Kerby who wanted Tom to hike with him in the Shenandoah Valley, a package with two rolls of developed slides from a sailing trip we took before Sarah was born. His mail remained unopened and unread. The note about the autopsy stayed in the growing pile of mail and messages that, as so many other things, were left undone during the strike.

In September, the strike ended; the hourly workers signed the contract as it was originally written. Management won. For four months, Tom and I had led almost separate lives. We faced each day and each evening without Sarah and without each other. Had the strike not kept Tom away from home 19 hours a day, I would have continued to follow him everywhere, to rely on him constantly; without him, I somehow learned to rely on myself. The paradox is that although Sarah's death made me dependent upon him, learning to live without her was a solitary journey for both of us. Years later, Tom told me that by working the strike and his regular job – a total of 19 hours a day – he, like me with my endless activity, worked through the initial, frantic, free-fall phase of grief.

14. The autopsy

I wanted to know the results of the autopsy, but I didn't want to see the neonatologist again. I wondered if Tom and I could hear the results from our regular pediatrician. I was shaking a bit when I called the neonatologist's office – not sure the secretary would release the report – but all she said when I asked her if she would send the report to our regular pediatrician was, 'Name and address of the pediatrician?' Two weeks later, Tom and I were called from the waiting room full of mothers, fathers, and babies and toddlers into the narrow hallway that led to the doctor's office. In the privacy of the hallway, tears that had been building for minutes and months surfaced. What would the autopsy tell us? Whatever the results, it would be about Sarah's painful death while I lay on the hospital bed waiting for the phone call from someone saying that she had arrived safely in Wilmington. Whatever the autopsy revealed, it would be about her ravaged body, the aftermath of an unchecked bacteria that could have been stopped by antibiotics before or after birth.

A nurse, one I'd seen many times in the office, scooted past Tom and me to put something on the doctor's desk. Seeing my tears startled her.

'What's the trouble?'

'We're here to get the autopsy results – from our baby's death,' I said.

'I know, but the tears?'

I couldn't begin to explain. 'It's a bad day,' I told her.

Tom and I sat across from the doctor while he flipped through the pages of the report and read: 'The cause of death was heart failure, yes, and, specifically, fatal arrhythmia brought on by sepsis, the blood infection. No congenital problems; her heart was normally developed. It also says she had a massive infection of the brain.'

He stopped reading out loud but continued reading to himself.

'The sepsis was caused by group B streptococcus, right?' I asked.

'Yes.'

'Does it say anywhere in the report if she was premature?'

'It says she was fully developed, full term. We had a couple of babies here a year or so ago who contracted group B streptococcus. They were pretty sick, but with antibiotics, they came around.'

'I wish you'd taken care of Sarah.'

PART 3

15. The aerobics class

When summer ended, the storm at sea still raged, but I was coming out of hove to after five months of denial, despair, and depression. I wasn't drifting anymore; I was angry and aiming for a number of targets. The odd thing was I didn't recognize my anger at first; someone else did. It all began unexpectedly during an aerobics class.

In the fall, I'd gone back to my job as a kindergarten aide at the same elementary school that Molly and Em attended. One morning, the voice on the intercom jolted the kindergartners into silence. 'Mrs Vigour, phone call. You may take it in the office.' The school secretary didn't tell teachers and aides about many calls – just the important ones.

Tom was on the other end of the phone. 'The doctor's taken a biopsy. We'll know the results in a day or so. The doctor was a little worried. My back is sore where he cut out a piece of the lump.' Stunned, I couldn't speak.

'Are you there?' Tom asked.

'Yeah.'

'I'll see you when I get home.'

We knew the lump was just a boil. The doctor would lance it, put a Band-Aid on it, and that would be that. So we hadn't worried. Now, I held the receiver for seconds or minutes while I tried to decide what to do with news like: having a biopsy done. And what to do with thoughts like: What if it's cancer? What if he dies? I noticed the school secretary looking at me. I said goodbye to the dead phone receiver and put it back on its hook on the wall. I walked out of the office dazed.

'Wha'd ya do, lose your best friend?' Miss Gibbs asked me in the hall between the teacher's lounge and the fourth grade rooms.

'Tom's having a biopsy. My God, I can't take anymore.'

She curved her large, fleshy arm around my shoulders and propelled me into the teacher's lounge, which was mercifully empty.

I heaved the words out between sobs, 'What if it's cancer?'

Her arms enclosed my sobs and my fear in a manageable package. 'Life's not gonna wait on you to finish grieving for that baby. It just goes on doing its own thing.'

Days later, Miss Gibbs said, 'Please say you'll take aerobics. If I can get three more people to sign up, I'll have enough for a class.'

'Aerobics? Why would I want to take aerobics? For you, I might just sign up. But I won't promise to stay in the class.'

'Try it, you might like it. It beats being a pressure cooker.'

'Who's a pressure cooker?'

'You, that's who. Tom's waitin' on a biopsy and you're blowin' a gasket.'

'You would too.'

'Don't get defensive on me. Just sign up for my class. It'll do you some good. Wasn't that biopsy supposed to be done by now?'

'Something got messed up at the lab. They had to take another slice of the lump. It will be a few more days before we know.'

'The class will meet in my room after school. Mondays and Thursdays.'

Miss Gibbs had a gift for teaching aerobics. The class lasted 45 minutes. During the first ten minutes, she had us swaying to slow dance music. Gently we'd reach, stretch, wiggle, and warm up. Then, to rock music, she'd lead, tease, and coax us into fast dance steps, jumping jacks, and high stepping or butt-kicking lopes around the kindergarten pod. 'Kick butt and knees to nose,' she'd holler and call out the names of those of us who moved too slowly or did not lift our legs high enough.

Finally, the slow music sounded the beginning of the end. Reward, she called it, for hard work. Floor exercises were slow and deliberate. Miss Gibbs, with humor and encouragement, would lead us through stretches that worked out every kink or cramp. One of her favorites was the fire hydrant. She had us on our hands and knees, then we'd lift one still-bent leg until it was parallel to the floor. With a quick movement, we kick that leg to straighten it out. The first five kicks didn't hurt, but by the 15th or 20th, we were in agony. Muscles that never had been used were ordered to stretch and contract and hold up one very heavy leg after another. The male dog's favorite leg lift was a challenge to us human females.

The morning after the first class, I was surprised to hear the alarm clock. In the five months since Sarah's death, I had not heard the alarm. I'd always wake before it went off. For the first time in five months, I'd slept for five hours. When I pulled at the sheet to cover my bare shoulder, my arm and chest screamed in pain. The pain ran around to my back. I tried pulling the sheet with my other arm. The same thing happened. I found that if I kept perfectly still, my arms, chest, and back did not hurt. I knew I had the flu. Nothing else could hurt this much.

I slipped one leg from under the covers and eased it to the floor. My leg would not support itself or my body. In one swift movement, I rolled from the bed to the floor. The impact did not hurt as much as the sensation of moving any part of my body. While lying on the floor, trying to figure out what was happening to me, I remembered the aerobics class. I didn't know I had so many muscles, and every one of them was screaming. Tom hooked my bra that morning because I could not make my arms bend back far enough to do it myself.

I did not know it then, but Miss Gibbs' aerobics class was the beginning of what was to become a lifelong addiction to exercise. I became addicted to the sleep I got after each aerobics class. After several nights of sleeping five hours at a time, I felt less like a zombie. I began to trust my mind to supply me with words and thoughts. I could open my mouth and an entire comment would come out. Before, sleepless, fitful nights robbed my mind of the ability to complete a sentence or a thought. I'd walk away leaving the words hanging, unfinished, unsaid.

The more I exercised, the less trouble I had with anxiety attacks that left me short of breath and frightened of crowds, frightened of being alone, frightened of stressful situations sometimes as minor as waiting at a four-way stop. *Will each person take his or her turn? Will someone go out of turn? Will someone run into my car? Kill my daughters? Or me?*

I signed up for another class. Tuesdays and Fridays from 5.00

to 6.00 p.m. I took an aerobics class at the city gym. The nights after aerobics classes, I'd sleep for five hours.

'Punch that bag,' Miss Gibbs called out to us students. 'You haven't moved the bag. Punch it harder. Get that bag to sway.'

We jabbed at our imaginary bags. It wasn't until we put all of our weight and all of our energy behind the punches that Miss Gibbs said she could see the bags just a swayin'. After punching class, a first grade teacher's aide told me that I looked angry as I jabbed. I didn't think I was angry until she mentioned it. But the more I thought about being angry, the more I thought that I was very angry.

I was furious at the neonatologist for not suspecting group B strep, the leading cause of death of newborns by infectious disease, and for blaming me for her death. He couldn't even tell me that she had died. He just stood there staring at me while my life, as I knew it, was gone. So, I said, 'She's dead.' And I asked why.

'You didn't come to the hospital soon enough,' he replied.

Going to the hospital sooner would not have changed the neonatologist's diagnosis, because neither he nor the obstetrician considered the possibility of a group B strep or any infection. By wrongly assuming that her breathing problem was due to prematurity, her life was over before it began. She was probably infected before she was born and could have lived only if I'd been given antibiotics during labor or if she'd been given antibiotics within hours of her birth. Studies and warnings and tests for group B strep were in the medical journals years before her birth, but the bacteria was not on many doctors' radar screens then. Doctors dodged the medical and legal issues of group B strep for nearly 30 years. If a mother's test for the bacteria was positive and the baby died, then the doctor was liable because he knew it was there; therefore, not testing served the doctors for a while. Treating had its own problems. Although 30–40% of women carry group B strep, only one or two of them will deliver babies who contract the bacteria. So to treat with antibiotics would be to treat 98 women out of 100 unnecessarily. It would be another decade and more before angry parents and frustrated doctors would mount a campaign that would put group B strep on all US obstetricians' and pediatricians' and neonatologists' radar screens and testing all pregnant women would become routine.

One of the nurses at the hospital told me the day Sarah died that the neonatologist changed hospital policy because of Sarah: Any pregnant woman whose membranes had ruptured for more than 12 hours was given antibiotics intravenously for the rest of her labor. But five months into grieving, the facts and answers I'd researched didn't soothe my anger.

After Sarah died, the nurse-midwife told me I was only thinking of myself. She had told me that she didn't want to be delivering my baby after midnight. Did she mean I was selfish because the baby came after midnight when she wanted to be asleep in the call room? I wondered if I should have gone to the hospital after the water seeped. Is that what she meant? Guilt is a huge part of grief, diminished only with the realization that some things are not in our control. No one in the hospital took any precautions to prevent Sarah from picking up an infection even though membranes had ruptured. My going earlier would not have helped Sarah which made the nurse-midwife's comment all the more callous.

I was angry that the hospital wasn't staffed with people trained to be gentle with someone who is grieving. Articles on grieving explained that thoughtless, cruel remarks by members of the hospital staff intensified grief. Why didn't someone from the hospital call Tom or my mother and ask them to be with me while Sarah was so sick and at the moment I learned she died? Why tell me that I had to take a tranquilizer, which I did not have to take. Why not ask me if I would like one. Taking a tranquilizer wouldn't have helped me to cope with the shock of Sarah's death. It might have helped the hospital staff. Subdued with drugs, I would not have been a bother to them. How could a nurse say that the hospital morgue couldn't keep the body after 10.00 a.m.? Why not explain that funeral homes are open 24 hours a day? I had never been in charge of a funeral before. I didn't know. Why didn't someone call Tom or my mother to tell either of them to do something with the body? A nurse told me, 'You can cry now.' She had a schedule for the course of my grief? She was giving me permission to grieve? Who granted her that right?

Yes, I was angry.

I wondered why hospitals are in the business of dealing with illness and death if the staff doesn't understand grieving? If birth cannot be respected and celebrated in a hospital, then why are hospitals in the business of birthing? Nurses and doctors, under the guise of hospital/doctor policy, interfered with so many natural instincts: when I wanted to hold my newborn babies, when I wanted to breastfeed them, when I wanted to look at them. How can such strong maternal needs be ignored by hospital staff? Why is hospital policy counter to mothers' instincts? And babies' needs? If laboring women go to hospitals for help should it be needed, why wasn't it there for me? When Sarah was born and the pain was unbelievable, the nurse-midwife did nothing to help. So what good did it do me to be in a hospital? The intense pain, I read later, was related to the group B strep; mine was not a normal delivery.

I was livid at parents who don't treasure their children. The news stories of newborn babies found in garbage cans made me weep.

I was angry that Sarah's death robbed me of the innocence that ignorance provides. I hated the stinging sensation of knowing that an accident or a disease can take Molly or Emily or Tom from me, and I might never see them again. Since Sarah's death, I hug Tom and my girls before they go to school or to a friend's house or to work and think, let me remember this moment always. It may be my last with her or him. It is not a sick thought or a paranoid one. It is a knowing thought. When loved ones die without warning, you know that you only have them today. There are no guarantees for tomorrow.

Yes, I was angry. That imaginary punching bag took thousands and thousands of hits before my anger dissipated.

I called my friend Anne, the nurse I'd asked to help me deliver Sarah at home. Considering the outcome, she must have been relieved that she had not assisted me with a home birth. Yet, maybe if she had, we would have seen that the baby was having trouble breathing and taken her to our regular pediatrician who would have started antibiotics immediately. Grief is filled with what ifs. Anne brought homemade chocolate chip cookies to Molly and Emily after Sarah died. She and her husband, Chuck, sat on the couch in our living room that first night I was home from the hospital and endured the awkwardness of wondering what to say and what to do. I loved them for coming because I, too, had felt awkward as I began a journey I never wanted to take as the new member of a club I never wanted to join.

I called Anne five months after she and Chuck brought the cookies and asked her what they teach nurses in nursing school that makes them unable and unwilling to be sensitive with a person who has just learned of the death of a loved one. I told her about the nurse who came into my room moments after Sarah died and told me I had to take a tranquilizer. Why do I need a pill if my baby has just died? And not just *a* baby, *the* baby I'd been trying to have for nearly three and a half years and after three miscarriages. *'Here's a pill.'* I asked Anne what they teach nurses and told her it certainly wasn't compassion, for Christ's sake.

Anne agreed but said nurses were taught survival – for themselves. She explained that they learn to distance themselves from patients' emotions, out of necessity. If a nurse were to allow herself to imagine the pain from the death of a child, or the emotional and physical pain of terminal cancer, how effective could she be? Anne asked. The patient would be crying and the nurse would be crying. This is supposed to be healthcare here not a support group. Nurses deal with death and pain every day. They must maintain a professional distance. That distance is what allows them to continue to do their jobs.

I asked Anne if nurses and doctors could distance themselves so much that they become cold to suffering. Are you just going to treat bleeding wounds and not broken hearts? Whatever happened to treating the whole patient?

Again, she agreed that healthcare means dealing with the whole patient. And she explained that there is a fine line between caring and caring too much. Nurses must first take care of themselves so that they are able to take care of others. Death isn't easy for anyone. Whether it is watching it happen, trying to prevent it from happening, or telling the family it has happened, she said.

I asked her if nurses are told to give tranquilizers instead of hugs. She said it wasn't an easy question to answer, and she didn't know the procedure at the hospital I was in, but she supposed that my obstetrician left standing orders to dispense mild tranquilizers to new mothers who are distressed. Say, a mother is having a hard time getting the baby to nurse or she's tearful over not being able to see her two-year-old who's at home. Situations like those could have come up so often in the past that the obs leave standing orders to dispense tranquilizers rather than have the nurse call him when he's asleep or beep him on the golf course or while he's in surgery. Anne guessed that I was not being singled out by being offered a tranquilizer.

Why would a nurse tell me I could cry. I didn't need someone's permission. A basic course in grief says that everyone's reaction is different, and the griever sets the pace, not a nurse or anyone else. Her answers began to come more quickly as if she had caught up to my pace, which was rapid as pent-up anger was unleashed. She began to piece it all together: my emotion, the doctors' and nurses' roles, and my need to come to peace with the lack of emotional care in the hospital.

She characterized the LPN on duty that night, suggesting that she was 22 years old, didn't have any children but wanted some someday. She had no training in grief or death and dying as none are required to get her license. She hadn't yet been able to attend a workshop or a seminar on 'The nurse's response to the mother whose newborn dies.' She was on duty the night a baby died at a small rural hospital where there was no money budgeted for social services or counselors and there was no chaplain on duty. It was her kindness and concern, all the characteristics that drove her to nursing, that propelled her down the hall to my room armed with nothing but a box of Kleenex. She ran into the room where no one else in that hospital wanted to be that night and said the only thing she could think of that might be helpful, 'You can cry now.' Anne told me I could direct my anger toward our cultural lack of ability to be compassionate with grief-stricken parents rather than the LPN with a heart.

When I asked Anne about the nurse who waltzed into my room saying, 'We can't keep the body in the morgue after 10.00 in the morning,' my anger showed as I said, 'She must be paid by the Department of Corpse-Free Morgues.' Anne said that some people have a knack for dealing with patients who are grieving, and this one apparently did not.

If doctors have more training in dealing with grieving people, why didn't a doctor counsel me, I asked. She said medical school reflected our culture, and neither does a good job dealing with or educating about grief. Like most other people-skills, experience is the teacher here, she told me.

The last issue I brought up was the biggest, the one I would wrestle with for years, the neonatologist. I told her the things he'd said to me in the hospital. Anne guessed that he sounded scared – not scared of me so much as scared of grief. She talked about the various responses to death: people wail, scream, hit themselves or nurses or doctors, faint, and/or become numb from shock. The neonatologist didn't know what to expect from me. I mentioned and Anne agreed that the neonatologist was not thinking about my grief so much as a possible lawsuit.

The phone rang after Anne and I finished talking. It was a nurse reporting about Tom's biopsy. Negative, she said.

16. Fragile connections

That fall Tom announced that we were going to church as a family. He didn't care if we went to a Catholic church or an Episcopal one, but we were going, starting Sunday. Catholic, I said. Then he asked if I would find out what time Mass starts or should he. I told him I would.

The decision to go to church as a family came from the man who snickered 'spectacles, testicles, wallet and watch' the first time he saw me make the sign of the cross. It came from the man who told me that God is not in a church. 'If there is a God, he's in the woods where I work.' It came, too, from the man, who on going to church with me the first time asked, 'You're not going to fill *our* house with all that crap, are you?' referring to the crosses, and statues, larger replicas of the ones in my mother's house. The same man who said we would start going to church regularly had balked but conceded to baptizing our daughters, saying he couldn't take a God or a religion seriously that thinks children are born with sin. Original sin? You've got to be kidding, he'd said. Tom, a scientist, a non-practicing Episcopalian, who believes in what he sees, had not been to church in a decade. But like me, he had wanted to have someone we could call to do the services for Sarah, someone we knew. Going to church was like buying insurance; if or when someone died, we would have a support system in place. It also became more than that.

In the years I hadn't gone to church, I hadn't stopped praying and receiving comfort or direction from the meditation, but physically going back reunited me with the rituals that had been part of my life for as long as I could remember. From that first Sunday and for the decades that followed we went to church as a family, just as Tom had said we would. As we restored our family that had crumbled under the stress of grief, the Sunday morning messages took on new meanings: be comforted and comfort others.

My cousin, Ann, called to say that her sister, Mary, was in the hospital and her new baby, Governeur, named for their father, was in intensive care because he had group B strep. The baby was given antibiotics soon after he was born.

'The doctors say he will be fine,' Ann said, but she also asked if I agreed. 'We now know how you felt when Sarah was sick,' she added.

'No, you can't know,' I told her. 'Your nephew will survive. Your worst fears will not become reality. Mine did.' Then, Ann, who is never at a loss for words, was silent. I thought I had come on too strong. But then I remembered that that wouldn't silence Ann. I realized she had called for sympathy. My experiences with Sarah should have enabled me to soothe her pain of having a nephew who was ill with group B strep. I told her that from all my research that the doctor was right; the baby would be fine because he was given antibiotics so soon after birth. The conversation left me full of pain and joy for Ann and Mary, and it took me back to living for 18 hours with my worst fears. I would be able to comfort others, especially grieving parents, but that fall, only five months into the grieving process, was too soon. I would remember that conversation and my reaction years later at a funeral. A former nurse to the child lying in the casket, was in a corner of the funeral home crying. I knew her husband had died a year earlier. I put my arm around her. She said she'd come to help and was disappointed in herself for crying. I told her that she'd be immense help to people, but later. A year into the grieving process is too soon; the wounds are too fresh to separate your hurt from others'. The wounds do heal enough to comfort, and bereaved parents offer comfort as only those who've buried children can.

That fall Kath dropped off some clothes that Molly had left at her house when she spent a night with her daughter, Lynn. She had only a few minutes to visit before she had to pick up her five-year-old, Tricia, from dance class. So Kath and I stood by her car in the driveway. I gazed at nothing. Kath, seemingly knowing what I was thinking said, 'It's good you didn't get to bring her home from the hospital. That way you didn't have a chance to get attached.'

I knew Kath meant to be helpful, but what is grief if not evidence of attachment? I wanted her to know where I was emotionally so we could stay connected, so I could bridge the gap between us, so I could explain and she would understand, and we could share experiences as we always had, so she could continue to comfort, so I said, 'I would give everything I own to hold her one more time.' Kath reacted with such a pained expression that I realized I shouldn't have said anything. At that moment I knew that we could not share the reactions or the range of emotions following the death of a child; words cannot bridge that gap.

My brother Pete came to visit on a Saturday when Tom had taken the girls to a pumpkin patch to find the best 'jack punkins,' as Emily called them. Molly, the sage, who couldn't let Emily's malapropism go by unnoticed, caught my attention and glanced toward the ceiling. She whispered that Emily meant jack-o' lampkins. 'You know, Mom: light, like a lamp.' She winked. I winked back.

I knew something was wrong when I saw Pete's face. His characteristic good humor, his happy-face smile wasn't. 'It's over,' he said, 'Cynthia and me,' and he slumped into the canary-yellow beanbag in the family room.

'The engagement?'

We didn't have any champagne in the house the evening he and Cynthia came to tell us they were getting married. The pictures we had taken months before were on the counter top in the kitchen. Tom, Cynthia, and Pete were toasting with champagne flutes half-filled with bubbly-red Cold Duck. Molly, Emily, and I were drinking grape juice. I was hugging Pete, and he was trying to hug back without touching the bulge under my brown and orange maternity top. The smiles in the pictures were so big that I expected to hear laughter when I looked at them.

Pete couldn't help noticing Cynthia, the beautiful, slim blonde at his high school. But it was her singing that sparked all that followed. She began singing with Pete and his friends, Mark and Les, in their band, *The Cuzins*. The band was booked regularly nights and weekends at local clubs. Pete, Mark, and Les, all gifted musicians, played guitars. In addition Pete played banjo. Their performances were more than a display of musical talent; they set each other up for jokes as well as solos. They'd change keys by reaching into pockets of their jeans and exchanging car keys. Audiences loved them. Then Cynthia started singing with them and audience-appreciation turned to adulation. 'She sings like an angel,' Pete told me after her audition. He tried to describe her voice to me, and then realizing there were no words, he pulled up the sleeves of his shirt to expose his goose bumps. 'That's how well she sings,' he said. Their engagement was part of a natural progression.

'What do you mean, it's over?'

'She's going to Texas.'

I knew that she was being courted by another band, but I never thought that that would interfere with the engagement. Pete didn't want to elaborate. He just wanted comfort. For a couple of hours, we talked or didn't. He sipped beer. I'd see him tear up and try to say something soothing.

I didn't know until then that empathy took energy I didn't have since Sarah's death. But after Pete left, exhaustion kept me from being able to move my arms and legs.

When I saw my little girls sitting too quietly, holding their Aceys, staring at nothing with hollow-looking eyes that peered from dark caverns, I was at once four and eight years old; I remembered that same loneliness after my brothers died. I moved to one then the other, reaching out, tenderly, willing them to let me love them again. For months their world had been shaken, their parents distant, and withdrawal had been a defense. 'May I hold you in my lap?' I asked Emily who nodded her head ever so slightly, hardly daring to hope for what she had known – for a mom whose attention had been as forthcoming and as necessary as warmth from the summer sun. 'My lap is big enough for two,' I said to Molly whose interest appeared to be on something outside the living room window. I put my arms around Emily's arms and cupped her thighs with my hands. We rocked in the rocking chair as she adjusted her body to form itself to the contours of mine. We spoke in the spirit-nurturing body language of skin and touch and warmth. Molly was by my side, her once-glazed eyes were reddened coming back to life. How many times in the past months had she needed her mom's hug and I hadn't noticed? When had I hugged her last? Her tears were those of abandonment and of daring to hope for what she needed. I scooped her into my lap and the three of us began to let go of what we had lost and to hold tightly to what we had.

17. Thanksgiving and Christmas

The first Thanksgiving without Sarah came fully laden with memories and buried hopes. No matter how we would have spent the holiday, it would have been difficult, because holidays and anniversaries are just a tough part of grieving. Grief comes in predictable and unpredictable waves that threaten to wash over its victim and carry her or him out to deeper and deeper water. Holidays and anniversaries are predictable waves. A year earlier we were happily expecting the new baby. As it happened Thanksgiving coincided with the end of the longest, loneliest, heaviest period of grief: the first six months. It was more like seven months in my case, but that's close enough. The end was much like a collision, but end it was.

We went to Virginia after two of our dear friends from college called early in November. 'Spend Thanksgiving with us, please,' Polly said. 'Come unload, grieve.' Unload, I thought, what a good way to put it. I could tell them everything: how it felt as if my skin had dissolved, the loneliness and the insanity of grief. Through it all, they would nod and say, 'Go on.'

'Of course we'll come,' I told her. 'Thank you for thinking of us. We need this. What can we bring?' I was overwhelmed by their kindness.

'Just bring yourselves,' Polly said. 'We are here for you.'

Something came to life within me after that phone call. Maybe because friends in our town seemed no longer sympathetic – as if I was supposed to be over it by now or they were weary of listening, or they didn't know what else to say. Tom and Polly were offering to listen, and I welcomed a new audience. By telling the story of Sarah again and again in the first year or two after her death, we were doing the work of grieving. Slowly it was becoming real, slowly our emotional selves were accepting the unacceptable, accepting what our intellects knew to be true.

Tom and Polly, an elementary school teacher, married years after my Tom and I did. Molly and Emily were toddlers when they married. Polly and I became friends after she had two emotionally and physically difficult miscarriages. I told her how tough it was for me to continue going to baby showers after miscarrying. She agreed. She understood how I lost touch with Judy, my best friend in grade school and junior high in Alexandria, Virginia. Judy wrote to tell me that she and her husband were expecting their first baby. Her letter arrived during the years I was trying to become pregnant for the first time. I never wrote back. It was hard to be happy for her when I wasn't sure I would ever become pregnant.

Polly's husband, Tom, combined his passions for medicine, architecture, and animals by becoming a veterinarian and designing and building additions to their home. He added a turret, a staircase off the master bedroom, skylights, a deck, and a sunroom. At last count Tom and Polly had three dogs, a cockatiel, and a ferret. One of the funniest people I know, Tom can weave a pun into a serious conversation lifting pathos to something giddy. I met him while we were in college at Virginia Tech. We became acquainted at a time when we were studying, dating, leaving home, pulling up old roots and not yet planting new ones, a time when relationships are marked by few pretenses.

I gathered presents for Tom and Polly, asked neighbors to care for the cat and dog and collect the mail, and packed for our trip 350 miles away. What Polly and Tom didn't tell us was that they were expecting their first baby in three months. My reaction at the sight of her already large womb was physical, as if I'd been hit in the stomach. I doubled over and thought I would vomit. Then I pretended to stumble and catch myself, so as to hide my reaction. The pregnancy was another surprise to my world that was listing, heeling, tilted over because of surprise. It would be a long time before we traveled again and dared to be in situations out of our control. I couldn't unload to Polly and Tom. I knew too well the vulnerability of pregnancy; I couldn't add to her fears or Tom's.

I never cried during the three-day Thanksgiving weekend, and I didn't tell my Tom; I was afraid to. I was afraid I wouldn't be able to stop crying. So I squelched my feelings; with no place to go, the hurt and anger swirled inside of me for three days, growing stronger as does a hurricane at sea.

After we said our goodbyes and drove away, I cried and I wanted my pain to be someone's fault. Tom was dumbstruck. He wanted to bask in the afterglow of a lovely weekend with old friends, savor the memory of lounging in their new hot tub with glasses of wine and laugh some more over the wine we brought. We could never trust the fellow at the liquor store to recommend wine again. 'Muscadine,' the man said running the tip of his tongue across his upper lip as if tasting something sweet and tangy. All while his eyes were closed in delicious reverence. 'Yep, we're fortunate to have such good, local wine,' he'd said so convincingly, with his eyes-closed-lip-licking, that we bought three bottles in a hay-lined, custom-made box. Each bottle tasted like another flavor of vinegar, and each bottle generated more laughter with louder additions of uproars and feigned retching. The funny thing was we drank all three bottles. I apologized to Polly even though she wasn't drinking because of her pregnancy.

'The wine really was awful,' I told her. 'I'm sorry.'

'No, don't be sorry, not at all,' Polly said. 'This was too fun.

Had the wine been good, we wouldn't have been able to laugh so much.'

'How could they have done this to me?' I asked my Tom in the car on our way home.

'There's not a mean bone in their bodies,' he said.

'How can you defend them?'

'They didn't think they were doing anything wrong.'

'They invited us to unload, to grieve. We couldn't. Not while they are expecting.'

'But the turkey, the homemade stuffing, clean sheets, cardboard turkeys for Molly and Emily to color and assemble. They both went to a lot of trouble to give us a good weekend.'

'Do you think I was set up? By asking us to come and pour out our sorrows about Sarah – by not telling us about the pregnancy, don't you think they were setting me up to fall apart?'

'I think that sounds sick.'

'It should have been my choice to spend this Thanksgiving with a pregnant woman or not. But they didn't give me that choice.'

'They didn't think about it that much. They just invited us to spend a fun weekend with them.'

'How could they not think? I'm a remnant of a tragedy. All I can do is put one foot in front of the other and breathe. I don't need anyone to make things more difficult because they aren't thinking or they just don't bother to warn me or ask me if I would like to spend a weekend with an expectant mother and admire the baby's nursery. My God, Sarah's only been dead six months.'

'Six months?'

'Yeah, six months.'

'No, six months' pregnant,' my Tom said. 'Polly got pregnant about the time Sarah died. They have been wrestling with this all this time. Trying to figure out how to tell us.'

'This is the way? Surprise!'

'It's not easy for them either. Think about it. You and Polly have been infertility buddies for years. Now, finally she's pregnant after we had Molly and Emily. Don't you think she wants to share this time with you?'

'I can't think about her feelings. I have too many of my own. It's more than Sarah; I may not ever have another baby.'

'I know this is tearing you apart. Everyone is sorry for you. There doesn't seem to be anything anyone can do. Even when someone does something, it is not right. Please don't cut everyone off. We're in this, too. You aren't the only one who's hurting.'

'It's not that I cut people off. It's more like no one we know has buried a child. It's difficult to talk with people who don't know what we are going through. Why can't I just hurt about this weekend without you asking more of me? I can't take anymore. It's not that I'm not happy for them. It's just all too painful to be around now. I know other people are pregnant and happy. I want that. I want another child so much it hurts. I can't share other people's pregnant joy, not now.'

'Do you remember when we camped on the Chesapeake Bay with Tom and Polly? Remember they came with us to the nature talk for kids? Remember when Emily ran to shake Smoky Bear's hand, and she was so little and so excited that she broke in line to be first? They were the only adults there without kids. They went just for us.'

'That's supposed to make up for this weekend?'

'No, it's supposed to remind us of who our friends are, and where they are coming from. Granted, they've never buried a child. They can't fathom what that is doing to us. But you can't blame them.'

'I wanted to feel better after this weekend, not worse.'

'Things happen. Like their pregnancy. They didn't plan for it to happen now. But they are trying to keep the door open, keep the friendship going, even though they are expecting and we are not.'

'It's easy to be friends with everyone when you're pregnant. You're happy.'

'Sometimes, I think you're so busy feeling sorry for yourself that you don't have any time or energy left to think of anyone else. It might do you some good to look at things from other people's perspective.'

'Oh, great. I'm grieving and I'm supposed to be considerate of other people.'

'Yeah. Something like that.'

'Your help I don't need.'

'I want you back. I want to see your smiles again. I want to hear you laugh again. I want to talk about anything else but how unhappy you are. I want to make love for fun not just because it's the right time of the month.'

'The girls will hear you.'

'They have their headphones on. They are listening to tapes.'

He found my hand and squeezed. I turned and looked out the window on my side. I had wanted his sympathy. I couldn't look at him, but I didn't move my hand away.

I wrote Tom and Polly a thank you note for the weekend without mentioning that their surprise news was difficult for me; no good could come from telling them that. Years later, we enjoyed fun weekends with them and their children and our children. I never did mention it. But I was changed by that weekend because I heard Tom nudging me to get a grip. If he had been nudging all along, I hadn't heard him, but on that drive home from Virginia I did hear him. Maybe I heard him because the first six months of grieving were ending, or maybe because I was jolted into the next phase by my friend's unexpected pregnancy. If it sounds unbelievable to not have heard Tom nudging me before that drive, it seems strange to me, too, but grief is powerful enough to have robbed me of hearing so I could heal. Only when I was able to begin thinking of him and the girls' feelings was I able to hear him. The cocoon was unraveling.

Between Thanksgiving and Christmas, I served each person's favorite food for dinner, every night. It started out as a thoughtful gesture: ham for Tom, taco for Molly, hot dog for Emily, but I couldn't think of what else they would like, so I just kept serving the same thing until Molly announced that she wouldn't eat another yucky taco and Emily agreed that she was sick of hot dogs, and Tom told them not to speak that way to their mother. And what sounded like a family feud was a good thing because I heard what each person said, and I was aware of the emotion propelling those words.

Later, Molly was stretched out on the living room floor watching TV, and I said that if she was finished drinking her Kool-Aid, she could bring me her cup because I was washing dishes. And she said, 'You're up. I'm not. You get it.' I wondered how could I be raising a child who would talk to me that way. So I repeated my request. 'Later,' she said, 'when the ad's on.' She was begging for boundaries, begging to be disciplined again. From the time she was a toddler, she had questioned the rules, challenged me to see if I meant business. And I assured her that *no* meant *no* always, over and over again. But then Sarah died and there were no boundaries, no rules, and anarchy reigned.

I asked Emily to pick up the pieces to her game and she told me she was too tired. So, I told her that tired or not, she was to pick up the game pieces. She had enough energy to take them out; she could put them back.

'No,' she said stomping her foot.

'Yes,' I yelled.

Then Molly whispered into Emily's ear and Emily said to me, 'Yeah, we do.'

'We do what?' I asked.

'Me and Molly hate you.'

And if it sounds like things were falling apart, they were, but the good thing was I was finally noticing. For seven months, my children were probably doing what they had just done – demanding to know their limits – to be in their safe zone where boundaries marked their world, but I had not heard them. When I did hear them, another phase of grief began: to rebuild what had collapsed. Tom and I talked about the decline in their attitudes and behaviors and decided on a three-part solution: they were not allowed to say yuck when food was served to them at dinnertime, backtalk was banned, and their allowance would be raised. The girls thought that adhering to the rules was a good trade for their new wealth.

I was beginning to admit to myself that I was part of a group I never wanted to belong to, and I wanted to connect with people who had buried children. There were no support groups for grievers in our small town, but I read in the state's newspaper, the *News and Observer*, of meetings in Raleigh for parents who had buried children who died of SIDS. There was also Compassionate Friends for grieving parents. The meetings were a two-and-a-half-hours' drive away, too far to drive on a weeknight. Then I read about SHARE, a support group for parents who had children who died during pregnancy or shortly after birth. There was no meeting place but an address was listed, so I ordered the newsletter from St. John's Hospital in Springfield, Illinois, and read that other parents suffer. I wrote letters; people from SHARE wrote back. One letter arrived that December. The woman told me of holding her newborn daughter, Elizabeth, while she died. I read the letter many times and came to realize that this mother was accepting the death of her baby.

In mid-December I walked by a church and heard organ music wafting through the open door. I gingerly peered inside. No one shooed me out, so I slipped into a pew in the back of the church and gazed at an altar full of singers in jeans and sweat suits. The choir director had stopped the organist and the singers to give directions. 'No hissing snakes,' he said. 'If you can't say "us" without hissing, then don't say the "s". Now, again,' the director said, raising his arms to the choir and nodding to the organist.

Born unto us a child is born
Unto us a son is given
Unto us a son is given
Born unto us a child is born
Born unto us a child is born
Unto us a son is given . . .
Wonderful, The Everlasting Father, The Prince of Peace.

One child, one wonderful child. Unto Tom and me a child was born – a wonderful child – and unto us that child was given and taken. I listened to the celebration of a child's birth in song, in chorus, in chant, in soprano and bass, through the organ and the choir director and Handel. I was supposed to be Christmas shopping, but for hours I listened to the celebration of the birth of a child and heard the heavens rejoice at each birth, each new beginning, each new life. They sang for Sarah.

Sarah would have been eight months old: crawling anywhere, everywhere, pulling herself to a standing position, grinning, babbling. It was the Christmas of what might have been – and the Christmas of the hamster.

Molly was eight and wanted a hamster. I told her that I pay an exterminator to get rid of mice that size, and I couldn't think about having a pet that looked like a mouse without a tail. She was not deterred. A hamster remained the first thing on her Christmas list. After reading that hamsters make nice pets, I told Molly, who was not yet ready to give up believing in Santa Claus, that although I would not buy her a hamster, she could ask Santa.

Under the tree Christmas morning, Molly found a red cage complete with an exercise wheel and a water bottle with a note: *To Molly from Santa*. The cage was empty. The golden hamster with white markings, the first hamster I had ever held, the one the pet store owner had told me was her best breeder, the one she parted with reluctantly, had raised the miniature wire gate and walked out of the cage.

'No problem,' I said. 'I read a book about hamsters. They are escape artists. Just think of little places they can get into. We'll find it,' I said trying to assure Molly and myself at the same time.

Molly was a mixture of emotions: happy about the hamster she was going to get and sad that it was not in its cage and, finally, as the family search went from minutes to a full hour, she became angry and tearful. I called my family to help. Pete came and found the hamster underneath the sofa in the living room. Although he had never touched one before either, I whispered to him that the lady from the pet store said it would not bite. He picked it up and handed it to Molly asking, 'What are you going to name it?'

'Kate,' she said.

I started to cry. Pete put his arm around me and propelled me out of the living room, so I wouldn't be crying in front of Molly and putting a damper on her happy time. 'If the next baby is a girl, I want to name her Kate,' I told Pete. 'She can't name her hamster Kate.'

Pete and Molly played with the hamster and discussed hamster names while Mom and I sectioned grapefruits and cooked scrambled eggs, fried potatoes, and toasted English muffins. Before sitting down to breakfast Molly introduced Tom, Emily, Grammie, Carl, and me to Hammy, short for Hamlet and kin to Hamster.

That Christmas, the pain of grief was back with an intensity I had not known in months. I thought I could concentrate on Molly, Emily, and Tom – and a hamster – and continue doing things with less deliberation, more naturally, not thinking about every move I made. But as the holidays arrived, emotions surfaced, emotions I thought I'd already dealt with. I cooked dinner for Tom, Molly, Emily, my Mom, Pete, and Carl. After we ate, my brothers offered to wash the dishes. Then, not knowing what to do with my sadness and realizing I was the only one unhappy, I put on my coat and told my family that I was going for a walk. When I left, I didn't know where I was going, but after I started walking, I knew. I walked to Sarah's grave, six miles away. I walked and cried.

The area where she was buried was much smaller than I'd remembered. I'd pictured more grassy area, more acreage. Other children were buried near by; I hadn't noticed any other graves or markers on the day of the funeral. I tried to imagine where our friends had stood. It seemed too small to have held as many people as had come. Some graves had stuffed animals or toys or flowers or balloons; others like Sarah's were unadorned. *Sarah Vigour May 3, 1981* was etched into the gravestone that tilted up a bit like a shim or a doorstop. The grave of a six-year-old girl from the elementary school where I worked was there; she'd just died of cystic fibrosis. I hadn't gone to the funeral; it was too soon after Sarah. I thought about the parents and where they were emotionally, and I realized how far Tom and I and the girls had come in eight months. We were beginning to accept the unacceptable. We were recovering.

The first Thanksgiving and the first Christmas were hurdles, but as with every first, the ones after were much easier until the pain no longer survived, only the memories.

18. Common ground

March wind blew gusty but warm enough so that I could stay outside and watch Tom while he changed the oil in his truck. I was sitting on the front porch steps when I heard the desperate squirrel.

'Have you ever noticed that sound before?' I asked him.

'What sound?'

'The squirrel. That pleading sound.'

'Oh, that,' he said. 'He's horny.'

'No, it's not a horny sound.'

'How do you know?'

'Horny is flirtatious. That is not a flirting sound. Listen. She is begging. That's a plaintive cry. She needs something desperately.'

'I'm telling you, he's horny.'

'It's a she. She needs more than a roll in the leaves.'

'What more could anyone need than a roll in the leaves?'

'Well, with an answer like that, I can tell you aren't a female squirrel.'

'And you are?'

'Oh, don't be silly.'

'You brought this up.'

'If you listen to that squirrel,' I repeated, 'you know she wants a baby. That's a mating call. Not for sex but for a baby.'

'Same thing.'

'It's the same thing if you're a man.'

'I thought we were talking about squirrels.'

'You just don't understand.'

'Maybe if I were a squirrel, I would understand.'

'Don't patronize me.'

He finished changing the oil in his truck and sat on the porch steps with me to watch the sun set as it only can set in the flat coastal plains – with the colors spread from street level on the left to street level on the right. Half the sky in blazing peach/pink, half the sky in pale blue-gray. Color and harmony. Be at peace, says God. Could there ever be peace again without Sarah? Before Sarah, squirrels chattered, teased, sassed, and were oh-so-nosey, now they are desperate. How could I not have heard that disturbing sound before? Tom moved closer until our thighs touched.

'Where do you suppose she is?' he asked.

'She is in the gum tree in DE Smythe's yard. See, to the right of his maple tree on that biggest branch? The fellow she's calling is across the street. Watch his tail flick. He isn't saying much back to her but his tail is responding.' The female chattered less. She cajoled less. But she was more active. She walked out on a limb and fanned her tail. The thin gray hairs spread a full and showy plume. The red flag had been waved. The male ran to the bending edge of a branch and leapt onto another one, closer to where the female was flicking her tail. In leaps and darts he moved closer and closer until she ran the other way. Either he ran fast enough or she stopped running, because, finally, they were spiraling up and down the same tree. The chase continued across a neighbor's lawn and out of view.

'I don't think I can make it without another baby,' I told him.

'We have two. Maybe it's time to accept that that's all we'll have.'

'I don't want the end to be a dead baby. "Oh, and how many children do you have?" Two and a dead baby.'

'But if we don't, have another, then what? What are you saying?'

'If I can't imagine having another baby, I can't go on.'

'You have Molly and Emily and me. Can't you be happy with that?'

'I know all that. But . . .'

He slid closer. Horny, I thought. Maybe he's right: what's the difference? Molly and Emily were having dinner and going to a movie with my mother. I took Tom's hand, stood up, and we walked into the house. Two weeks later I was gloriously, joyously, albeit guardedly pregnant.

The pregnancy didn't prevent my apprehension as the anniversary of Sarah's death approached. I took the anniversary day off as a personal-leave day from work because I was afraid I would cry at school. I tried to keep busy that day by doing laundry, vacuuming, sweeping off the deck, picking up toys, but my busyness didn't prevent the tears. I hadn't cried daily in five months, but I cried off and on that day for what should have been. I was sitting at the dining room table that May 3 holding wads of Kleenex in my fists when Tom came home from work. He held me close to him while I sobbed and told him that this baby probably wouldn't have red hair. He kissed my forehead, my hair, and whispered, 'This baby, boy or girl, will be a new person with its own personality and black or blond or red hair. The baby won't be Sarah, but she or he will be our gift to ourselves.'

Two weeks later a sharp, continuous pain woke me. It was unlike any pain I had ever felt. There was no throbbing, no ebb and flow, no relief. An obstetrician was called to the emergency room after a nurse checked me. He said only part of the placenta had torn away from the uterine wall. After 45 continuous minutes of nausea-inducing pain, the sensation stopped as abruptly as it began. The obstetrician thought there was a good chance the pregnancy would make it. He said I was to lie flat in bed in the hospital.

For three days, I never used a pillow. I learned to sip coffee through a straw, eat scrambled eggs with a spoon, talk on the phone, listen to the TV without seeing the picture – all completely flat on my back. Nurses sponge bathed me. Glenda, Kath, and Vera came to see me. Since I was lying flat, their faces would be inches from mine as they told me some news or a joke. The nearness and the angle of their faces made the jokes funnier. Then without warning, bleeding started heavily and didn't stop. The fetus spontaneously aborted, the bleeding continued, and the doctor ordered a D and C.

The tears were different this time. Lying on a stretcher outside of the operating room, I was alone but I was not lonely, just consumed by sadness. 'Someone will be along shortly,' said the orderly who'd pushed the stretcher from my hospital room as he locked the stretcher's brakes and left me in the cinder block hallway in the basement outside the operating room.

I could raise my head now, there was no need to continue lying flat. I looked around, and seeing no one, I laid my head down again and allowed myself to cry. Warm, wet tears spilled over my temples and into my hair, baby tears. I wasn't afraid of these tears as I had been of the ones that flowed after Sarah died. After Sarah, I was terrified of crying, afraid I would never stop, afraid the tears would control me, afraid I would drown in them, afraid

I would drown my family. But not these tears, not this baby. Grief was not fearful then, just oh, so sad.

I was giddy when I awoke after surgery. I didn't know that a D and C could do wonders for a person's mood. The obstetrician came to my room to tell me that everything went well, that I could go home the next day but not go back to work for a couple of weeks, and I was to take a nap every day. I'd lost a lot of blood, he said, and that was apt to make me tired. On his way out the door, he added, 'Oh, I put something in your IV to perk you up. You seemed down before surgery.'

Put something in your IV to perk you up? No, he cheated me of this time to grieve. What could he know about grief? If ever there was a time to grieve, it was now. A dead baby and five miscarriages entitled me to be sad before a surgery that would scrape out the remnants of another much-wanted pregnancy.

Soon the effects of the 'something in my IV' wore off and I plunged into melancholy. But this time, Glenda, Kath, and Vera, and I were on common ground. They, too, had had miscarriages. With the blood loss, I was extremely tired for weeks.

'To be expected,' the obstetrician said. 'Don't push yourself.'

I called Glenda. 'I'm so tired and weepy', I said.

'Part of miscarrying,' Glenda said. 'It happened to me.' She explained that her doctor said that the hormones that maintained the pregnancy stopped abruptly. 'I think it's the sudden change that wreaks havoc with our emotions.' Not to say that a miscarriage isn't reason enough to wallow, it's just that the sadness seemed out of proportion to the loss of a three-month fetus.

Trying to cheer me up, Glenda said, 'It won't last forever. Look, you've been talking about wallpapering the girls' room. Let's do it. It will give you a lift.'

Glenda spread wallpaper paste on a wall in Molly and Emily's room, smoothing over rough spots and filling tiny holes with paste, making the old wall look unmarred. She fanned her trowel easily, quickly, deftly. I dabbed my eyes with Kleenex and told her how miserable I was not to be pregnant. Just as easily, quickly, deftly, she tempered my tears by relating her experiences with miscarriage.

'I can't tell you how many times and how much time I spent crying after losing that baby', Glenda said. 'Now I think, if that pregnancy had continued, I'd have four children. Four. Thank you, Lord. Three is plenty.'

Kath brought Kentucky Fried Chicken and biscuits and made

a green bean casserole and tossed a huge salad. She and her girls, Lynn and Tricia, and her husband, Craig, ate with us that summer, a little more than a year after Sarah died. Vera brought roast beef. She had marinated it in a garlic sauce and cooked it, rare, over her grill. I don't remember which was better: seeing her or tasting the roast beef. For two weeks, teachers at school prepared meals and brought them to our house.

It seemed as if everyone I knew had had a miscarriage. For the first time in a year, I could exchange emotions with friends. That communion, that common ground, the sharing of experiences was to me like rejoining the world. My reactions were validated and because they were, I wasn't solitarily confined to grieve for the miscarriage as I was with Sarah. I was part of my friends' lives again.

19. A vacation from grieving

'It is important to remember you are not abandoning a dead child by laughing. It's all right to enjoy life. That does not mean you have forgotten your dead son or daughter. This is a very difficult truth for bereaved parents to accept.'

Dr Joseph Fischoff (Chief of Psychiatry, Children's Hospital of Michigan)

A month and a half after the miscarriage, we took our first weeklong family vacation in more than a year. We camped in the spacious, park-like, back yard of two of our closest friends from college, Doug and Karen, and made day trips to the 1982 World's Fair in Knoxville, Tennessee. Doug and Karen, their two sons, and daughter laugh. They joke with contagious abandonment. They laughed that week until I did, too, taking a holiday from grieving. I hadn't finished the work of grieving after the miscarriage and was only one-third to one-half way through the two to four years it takes to process the death of a child. I didn't realize then that there are no holidays from grieving. Grief waited for me.

One day at the fair it rained so unexpectedly that we were caught without raincoats or umbrellas, and it rained so heavily that Molly, Emily, and I held hands because we couldn't see each other through the downpour. We ran to a women's bathroom. Tom took shelter in a men's. Within 15 minutes, the worst of the storm was over, but it was still raining. Molly, Emily, and I wanted to leave the crowded bathroom, but we didn't want to get wetter. I saw a box of garbage bags and grabbed three.

'Mom, are you stealing?' Molly asked.

'No, our entry fee includes a bag each,' I lied.

I bit open the sides to make armholes and poked holes for our faces. I pulled the bags over Molly and Emily's heads as if I were slipping a pillowcase over a pillow. They came nearly to the ground. The rainbags were perfect for walking in the light shower and finishing our day at the fair. I put on my bag and grabbed one for Tom. Holding hands so we wouldn't slip on the wet cement walkways, we headed for the men's bathroom. I hoped officials at the fair wouldn't say anything to me for taking the garbage bags. Maybe we wouldn't be noticed, I thought.

A little girl tugged at her mother's shirt to get her to look our way, 'Mommy, look, those trash bags have feet!'

I walked faster to get out of her sight.

'Mommy, those bags are walking!' the little girl said again, pointing at us.

How much can I be charged for stealing four garbage bags? I wondered. Soon the little girl's excited shouts were heard by the people around us. They cleared a path for us. Mothers, fathers, brothers, sisters, couples, a Boy Scout troop stood in rows four people deep watching us bags walk. Maybe they thought that, like the robots at the fair, we were part of the show. When I looked up to see if we were still headed in the right direction, I saw Tom aiming his camera at us from the porch of the building that housed the men's bathrooms. Within 30 minutes, we had started a fad. Two-thirds of the people at the World's Fair were wearing garbage bags.

When we came back from the fair that day, we told Doug and Karen and their children about the rainbag fad. They ran with it, embellishing, asking to hear parts of the story again and retelling scenes in their own words until their renditions were better than the event itself. We laughed, the delicious roll-your-head-back kind, until our sides hurt.

When we got home our year-old cat, Harley, was sick and

after a ten-day illness had to be put to sleep. My brother Carl and his girlfriend had given us the long-haired black kitten after Sarah died. Molly and Emily named him after their Uncle Carl's motorcycle. 'I can't watch him die,' I told the veterinarian. 'He's having trouble breathing.' Then I told him about Sarah having trouble breathing. I cried noisily in front of the veterinarian, out of character for me, an introvert. The vet was most sympathetic. 'I understand,' he repeated. He stood patiently listening to my story as if there were no other animals or owners in his waiting room who needed his expertise.

I couldn't take Harley for his last trip to the vet myself. I called Kath; she drove the cat and me in her car to the vet's office. She took him inside while I sat in the car and cried. I am not even very fond of cats. I didn't know why I was taking Harley's death so hard.

Oddly enough, the problem was laughter, that *holiday* from grief. The week with our friends was an uproariously funny time, but it cost me emotionally. It reminded me of laughing with Tom and Polly that first Thanksgiving and plunging emotionally, afterward, and it disconnected me from Sarah. As long as I grieved for Sarah, I felt connected to her. If I laughed, I severed that connection maybe because I was doing something fun without her. Maybe by laughing I was going on with life and she was not. The aftermath of those first times of joyous laughter with friends was followed by sadness, a letting go, a necessary step in the process of getting on with the rest of life.

20. The birthday party

That fall, after school had started, but before Halloween, my mother's sister, my Aunt Pat, called from California. Aunt Pat, the businesswoman, said, 'T, your cousin Katherine has a hunch that something good is happening to you.' Katherine is psychic. She has never missed. When she has a hunch that something good is happening to someone, it is. Always. 'So what is your good news?' She laughed until I could picture her mouth open wide, her chin thrust forward, her eyes inviting. She laughed as if she knew the punch line, as if she'd set me up, as if I could end her story, as if we both could win. Aunt Pat is a glorious contradiction. She is all business and she is all Irish. She is a sculptor, an activist, a painter, a writer, a comedian. Her 11 children chisel a no-nonsense, business-woman exterior out of a passionate Irish/artist mold.

What could I say? Of course I thought baby. I was always thinking baby. But it was too early in the month to know. 'I don't have any good news yet, Aunt Pat,' I told her.

Irish passion, either up or down, was down when Aunt Pat sighed into the phone, a sigh of sadness for me and for herself. We are connected by our joys and by our griefs; it makes us family and friends. I couldn't respond by saying: I hope I'm pregnant. I always hope I'm pregnant. And I didn't want to start another avalanche of calls from relatives wanting to know if it was true. There had been so many false alarms with five miscarriages. I couldn't say anything until I had something more certain than hope.

'But Katherine is right here. And she is having such good vibes about you. Something must be happening.'

I told Aunt Pat that I'd let her know when I knew something. I smiled hanging up the phone, encouraged by Katherine's good vibes.

A week later, my temperature remained elevated. A home pregnancy test confirmed the thermometer readings. Even knowing what can go so horribly wrong at any stage of pregnancy, goose bumps erupted on my arms, as I was transported by hope, imagining all that might go well.

The obstetrician, the one the nurse-midwife who delivered Sarah worked for, agreed to screen me for group B strep throughout the pregnancy. The first culture, at seven weeks, was negative. Month after month, as the pregnancy progressed without incident, fears began to subside. Molly and Em gave up the lowest drawer of the toy cabinet in the family room for the baby; we filled it with baby rattles, cloth books, the brightly colored pop beads about the size of hen's eggs. We wiped the cradle's walnut wood of dust and washed the cradle's sheets that my mother had made, and we marveled at how a little joy can spread until it fills every room, every closet, and every cell of once-crushed hearts. As the last miscarriage had brought me back to common ground with my friends, that pregnancy brought me back to a life with hope.

I was six months pregnant when Emily turned seven. As a celebration of her birthday, and as it developed, a coming-out event for our family – as we hadn't had any parties in a year and a half – we invited neighbors and friends and family to a backyard carnival party. The games and activities were like those on a circus midway. Vera's and Steve's daughter, Jena, was the first guest to arrive. She carried a present half as big as she was. Her black hair was pulled back and tied with a bright pink ribbon that matched her pink and white corduroy jumper. She wore white tights and black patent leather shoes.

'Oh, Jena, what a big box,' Emily said trying to hug her and the box. 'What is it?'

'You have to open it to find out,' Jena said.

'Not yet,' I told Emily. 'Present-opening time is later. Can you girls guess how many chocolate kisses are in the jar in the living room? The winner gets to keep the kisses.'

Jena and Emily took off running.

Scott, Angela, and Michael – Glenda's and Tony's children – arrived next. Tom handed each of them a book of tickets and showed them the way through the gate to the backyard carnival. Soon Lynn, Tricia, Anita, Diana, and Donnie came. Last to arrive was Annette's boy, Corey.

'Corey, did you guess how many kisses are in the jar in the living room? Did you put your name and the number on a piece of paper? Did you drop the piece of paper in the box?'

He nodded and told me what a good guesser he is.

Molly was sulking. She was having a tough time watching her younger sister get all the attention. I told her that her birthday would be in just three months, and she was not to ruin her sister's party. After that, I ignored her, not giving attention to the understandable and human reaction of a slighted eight-year-old.

The partiers used their tickets to buy chances to win goldfish or have their fortunes told, or have their faces painted, or do the hero climb up a tall ladder to get a Tootsie Pop. Tom's father, Papa, set up a drawing booth. His homemade spirograph, a mechanical Rube Goldberg-like device, spun and twirled a mechanical arm that held colored pens. The pictures the spirograph drew were multi-colored geometric shapes that resembled the graphs of math problems that Papa does for fun.

My mother was in charge of the goldfish. For one ticket, a child could throw a ping pong ball three times into a cluster of fishbowls. If the ball landed in a fishbowl, she or he won the fish and the bowl. I told my mother that she could keep any leftover goldfish. She'd placed the ten flared-sided glasses close together. How could anyone miss?

'Party favors,' my mother shouted, hawking her wares. 'Get your goldfish party favors here. Everyone's a winner.'

For two tickets, Angela, Glenda's 12-year-old, painted butterflies and hearts on the girls' faces. The boys asked for pictures of skulls and crossbones. The children were so proud of their painted faces that they would not rub or scratch their cheeks even after the paint dried and their cheeks itched. Jena, whose father owned a sailboat like ours, asked Angela to paint a sailboat on her cheek.

'All our tickets are gone, Mom. Can we open presents now and blow out the candles and eat cake and ice cream?' Emily was asking.

'Sure, but not all at once,' I told her.

Soon wrapping paper covered the dining room floor. The dining table was littered with paper plates with half-eaten pieces of chocolate cake with pink icing, melting strawberry ice cream and unused napkins. Giggly children were holding their plastic 'fishbowls' and bags of favors while goldfish with vertigo bobbed up and down. I opened the front door so I could watch for mothers as they pulled into our driveway.

'Mom, this is the happiest day of my whole life,' Emily said before falling asleep. She was lying in her bed with all of her birthday presents around her. Under her arm was a large taupe-colored, floppy-eared bunny rabbit from Jena. She said it reminded her of the wallaby she and Jena had seen at the petting zoo. She also got a book of silly and fun poems by Shel Silversteen, *Where the Sidewalk Ends*, a Barbie doll dressed in a bride's dress, pink lipstick and a nail polish to match, ball and jacks, new red shorts with pockets and a T-shirt with hearts on it. Cuddling her new bunny, Emily said, 'I wish Sarah could have come to the party.'

'Me too.'

As sensitive as she is, maybe Emily said that for my benefit. Maybe she knew I'd spent most of the last year and a half thinking more of Sarah than of her. Maybe she remembered that Sarah's death had deprived her of a year and a half of a loving mom, of her normal homelife. Maybe she thought that if Sarah were there that her world would not have been turned upside down. Maybe she thought she could wiggle further into my heart by mentioning Sarah.

Molly was sitting on the couch in the living room. The room was dark. No lights were on. The television was not on.

'Something got you down?' I asked her.

'It's not fair that Emily's birthday comes before mine.'

'You're right. It's not fair.'

'I have to wait three months till my birthday.'

'We can't change your birth date. So, you have two choices. You can accept the fact that your birthday is three months after Emily's or continue to be unhappy.'

'It's not easy to accept.'

I scooted closer to her and put my arm around her slumped shoulders. 'We could start talking about the kind of party you'd like.'

'Swimming. At the sailing club. And I want more friends than Emily so I can get more presents,' she said, straightening her shoulders and becoming animated as she waved her arms around imaginary presents.

'Sounds like a good party to me,' I said, feeling relief that she could express her frustration at seeing her sister as the focal point of the day and that I could respond, that I could nurture again. I even heard Tom whistling in the backyard as he put up the ladder for the hero climb. This pregnancy, this baby – even before its birth – was giving us back something we had lost.

When I saw the obstetrician for the seventh-month prenatal visit, we discussed care for the baby after the delivery. Neither of us brought up the neonatologist, the one who cared for Sarah, and remained the only neonatologist at the hospital. The obstetrician suggested a general practitioner, an older man, semi-retired who wasn't taking new patients, but at the urging of the obstetrician, he said he would meet me. The obstetrician also assured me, to my relief, that he would be there when the baby was born, as his nurse-midwife was no longer working with him. Also, he asked me to fill out some forms at the hospital. The hospital's admitting nurse asked if I would want the neonatologist to be consulted should any problems arise. I told her no. Without the neonatologist and the nurse-midwife and with negative tests for group B strep, I approached the last two months of pregnancy with confidence.

The general practitioner was short and round. The hair he had left collected above his ears in reddish, gray tufts of curls. Sun had freckled his fair skin and his pink cheeks appeared to blush as he shook my hand. He had a smile but it was slight and shy, in fact, I wouldn't have noticed it at all except that as he turned his head to the side, I, too, turned mine and caught the barest upturn at the corners of his mouth. When I started talking, his shyness vanished, and he looked at me not with his head turned sideways but straight so he could hear my every word and its nuance and absorb every one of my facial expressions with his soft green eyes.

As I told the general practitioner about Sarah, he said, 'Poor Bob,' over and over as I related the story of her birth and death. Lines formed on his forehead in sympathy. I thought about telling the doctor that the neonatologist had no feelings for Sarah or me, so there was no need to feel sorry for him. But I didn't. I thought about reminding him that I was the mother in this sad story, but I decided not to. I decided that the general practitioner had not buried a child and couldn't relate to me, but if he'd had a patient who'd died, he could relate to the neonatologist.

Then, with emotion and concern equal to what he had shown the neonatologist, he said, 'Please, call me when labor starts. I would like to see this baby as soon as it is born.' Never had I known a baby doctor who wanted to know when labor started so he could see the baby when it was born. Any injustice I had felt when the general practitioner said, 'Poor Bob,' was obliterated when he showed such concern for my yet-to-be-born baby.

The obstetrician decided to induce labor five days past the due date, since I had developed gestational diabetes when I was seven months pregnant. The diabetes concerned the obstetrician, and he reminded me at those last few visits, 'We don't know why babies of diabetic mothers die sometimes, but they do. They die toward the end of pregnancy, suddenly and unexpectedly.' I didn't dwell on thoughts of burying another baby. Perhaps it was hope, or need, or the blessings we'd received as a family by this ever-growing womb, but I wasn't bone-chilled scared as I thought I would be with words like: 'We don't know why babies of diabetic mothers die; they just do.'

With the baby kicks' assurance of life, and without amniotic fluid leaking, and without contractions, the morning of the baby's birthday was calm; it was another doctor's appointment. While I rinsed our two coffee cups and four cereal bowls, juice glasses, and spoons and put them in the dishwasher, Tom took Molly and Emily to my mother's house. He was carrying his camera when he came back.

'How about a shot of you wiping the kitchen counters on the baby's birthday?' Tom asked.

'Forget it. You're not taking my picture. Not when I'm this big. Take some of the baby and me after it's born.'

'I can see it now: before and after shots – on the same day,' he said kissing the back of my neck.

'The answer is still no.'

'Is this a great day to have a baby or what?' he said, nibbling my ear.

'Let me guess. You're proposing the or-what?'

'There's still time.'

'There is not.'

'Then how about that picture?'

The picture shows me standing on the front porch holding the strap of my overnight bag in one hand and my purse in the other. He caught me with an embarrassed grin, but the bulging womb under my light blue, A-lined style dress overpowers all.

'This one will be captioned: *7.00 a.m.*,' he said.

It was warm and sunny the second day of June two years after Sarah. Flowers were blooming, grass was greening, gardens were sprouting; I could enjoy it all on the drive to the hospital without contractions to distract me. Tom and I caught up on business. Yes, my mother would make lunches for Molly and Emily, and cut up Emily's apple into slices because her front tooth was loose, and take them to school by eight in the morning and pick them up after school. Yes, most bills were paid. The ones that were not could wait until the next paycheck. We run out of milk every other day. The company that delivers salt for the water softener will not leave the salt without a check. Just clothespin a check to the water softener in the morning. We run out of milk every other day, but I should be home tomorrow if all goes as planned.

'You already told me about the milk.'

'I did? Oh, you're right. I did. I guess I'm nervous.'

'You're brave, you know, having another baby,' Tom said, putting his right hand on my knee.

'I couldn't have done it without you,' I said, reaching my hand to squeeze his.

'I would hope not.'

'Plus, I didn't like the alternative,' I told him.

'We're set on baby names, right?'

'Right. Mark or Kate.'

We talked about my brother Pete's wedding just five days earlier on the baby's due date, May 28. Pete's wife, Rhonda, finished the forestry technician program at the community college while making time to plan an elegant ceremony highlighted by roses, her satin gown, her romantic curls, and their smiles. They left the reception for Busch Gardens in Virginia where Pete had a summer job playing guitar. After that, they would be going to Boston where Pete would finish his degree in professional music concentrating on jazz guitar at Berklee College of Music.

Soon after we arrived at the hospital, a nurse came into my room and said, 'Your baby's doctor wants to know how you are doing?'

'Tell him I'm doing fine. And tell him not to come to the hospital yet. It will be a while before I have this baby. I haven't even been induced yet.'

About every hour, a nurse would come into my room to say that the doctor was on the phone and ask what to tell him about labor's progress. I basked in the attention from the *expectant* general practitioner.

'Tell him I'm about four centimeters dilated. It will be at least two more hours.'

Soon I saw the doctor's flushed cheeks in the window of the labor room door. His green eyes were bright and smiling with hope. He waved, but I was too busy to wave back.

A nurse took vaginal, nasal, and rectal smears, to start growing cultures to test for group B strep. If the baby got sick, he would know what the problem was and be able to treat it right away rather than wait for cultures to grow evidence of disease. He knew that I could colonize group B streptococcus at any time. Negative cultures throughout the pregnancy were no guarantee that I was not carrying the bacteria at the time of delivery.

Labor, even induced with pitocin, simulated natural labor until the dose was increased, and, oddly, I started crying between contractions. When the obstetrician came to check on labor's progress, I asked him to cut back on the pitocin. He obliged with a guarded statement about his wanting me to move along. I assured him that I can progress but I didn't need the tears. Having nasal swabs taken from the back of my nose hurt and made concentration on Lamaze difficult. The nurse would not wait until a transition contraction was over. But, I was able to regain control and handle the remaining contractions of transition – the shortest but most difficult part of labor. When the time came to push, I was frightened that I would again experience the pain I had felt pushing when Sarah was born. The obstetrician hadn't been there; he didn't know that all the Lamaze training didn't work when it came time to push Sarah. So he grinned and told me to push as if I would be relieved. I froze.

'What's wrong?'

'I'm afraid to push. It hurt so much the last time.'

'It won't now,' he said injecting a local painkiller.

It was quiet in the labor room, almost respectful. No one asked if she and her friends could watch. Tom and the obstetrician were there timing contractions, watching, encouraging, waiting. The baby's doctor paced the hall outside of the labor room. A labor room nurse handed the obstetrician utensils and prepared a warm bath for the baby.

The wetness and warmth of a tiny body slid against the inside of my right thigh. I heard a strong cry. The obstetrician handed the slippery red bundle to Tom, and I looked away.

'She's beautiful,' the obstetrician told me.

'I haven't been able to look at babies for two years.'

'You can look now.'

All my confidence dissolved. If I looked, I'd fall in love with her. If she was panting, or deformed, or heart damaged, if she were to die, I'd be better off not to have seen her. So I watched the obstetrician's face and Tom's. There was no sign of alarm. Their bodies were relaxed. Their expressions were more like wonder or awe.

The general practitioner didn't wait for an invitation. He was there in the labor room examining Kate. I studied his face and watched the movement of his arms from his shoulders to his elbows. I didn't dare look lower, not yet. He touched her all over, listened to her heart with his stethoscope, and finally grinned at me and nodded.

Tom handed her to me. I held her but still looked at Tom. He took a picture of the baby and me and captioned it: *5.00 p.m.* When I did lower my head to see Kate Bancroft Vigour, my tears made her a blur of arms, legs, tummy, toes, fingers, and a scrunched-up crying face. She had everything she needed and everything I needed.

Kate did not develop group B strep nor did she have any problems from my gestational diabetes.

Kate and I spent that night in the hospital. The next morning before Tom, Molly, and Emily came to pick us up, the neonatologist walked into my room grinning as if he were making a social call. I was in the bed, sitting up, propped up with pillows, holding Kate in my arms. At first I didn't recognize him, as I hadn't seen him smile before. When I did recognize him, I looked at him and his grin and assumed, and then hoped, that he had entered my room accidentally. He didn't speak. I had either too much to say to him or nothing at all. I chose nothing. In the fleeting minute or minutes that he was in the room, my facial expressions must have shown the blank stare of nonrecognition, and then of realizing who he was. He would have seen the look on my face when the flashback started, when I saw the light from behind him make his body a faceless silhouette as I thought of the last time I had seen him, those moments that altered the course of my life. I thought of the struggles of the past two years and how easily they could have been prevented if only he had given Sarah antibiotics. I thought of his misdiagnosis and his arrogance. His grin disappeared. I looked away. I heard the door close gently as he left.

Soon Tom, Molly and Emily came, and the girls dressed Kate in a clean diaper, a new yellow dress, and matching yellow blanket. Each told the other how to button buttons or pull the diaper's tape snugly. Something began that day in that hospital room, something about a family needing a baby and getting one.

21. Sail the wind

That first summer with Kate and the second one after Sarah, Roberta from the sailing club asked if I would like to teach a course with her: novice sailing for women. We used our boat, *The Molly Em*. At the beginning of the first class, I was so nervous I was shaking. I caught Roberta's eye and made motions to her to take the lead, be the head teacher. 'It's your boat,' she said, deferring to me, putting me in charge. Though I was an accomplished sailor, grief had taken its toll on my confidence. So there I was that first evening watching five women look at me as if they were out for an evening of entertainment. Roberta just smiled at me as if to say: What next skipper?

The one thing good about that evening was the wind; it was steady, not too strong but strong enough. Had the wind been lighter that first night out, sailing might have seemed too easy, and the women might not have been wary enough of the wind's strength and the need to compensate for it. My new students watched me motor out of the slip, hoist the main sail and the jib, and tie the reefing lines, that is roll the sail up around the boom to the first row of tie downs. Reefing the sail reduces the sail area and lessens the ability of the boat to point or steer close to the wind, but reefing also made the boat easier to handle. I kept thinking: They trust me, but do I know enough to be showing them anything? The confidence I lost to grief was regained one task at a time as I became a new me after Sarah.

I noticed a ripple in the water at the front, bow, of the boat indicating that the bow painter, the line used to tie the boat to the pier, was trailing in the water. Before heading to the fore deck to retrieve the line, I asked the woman next to me to hold the tiller and mainsheet. 'Here, take these for a minute while I get that line,' I told her. Her hands remained at her sides. Her eyes were big and startled. 'Have you ever taken the tiller and the mainsheet before?' I asked. She shook her head. My fear ended when I saw hers.

I was catapulted into teacher-mode, guiding them as my father had guided me when I was seven, more than a quarter of a century earlier. I'd watched my father snap the tiller into place, step the mast, lower the dagger, then raise the sail of his 14-foot Sailfish and zip into the Chesapeake Bay and back. I knew he was either a magician or a genius. He'd turn his face into the wind, and his black hair would blow back and his grin would be wider than I'd ever before seen. I was eager to learn to sail, so I could know his joy and share it with him.

During the first few years Tom and I were married, we'd lived in inland states, so when his company offered him a promotion that would take us to the coast of North Carolina, I was eager to move so I could sail again. We bought a 12-foot Minifish, much like a surfboard with a sail. As I showed Tom and Molly and Em the tricks and the absolutes of sailing as my father had shown me, I would hear my father's words. With every tug on the mainsheet, I'd hear his encouragement, his excitement at the strength of the wind and the hull speed and my boat handling. Tom and I and the girls had such fun darting from shore and back that we wanted to sail farther and stay out longer, so we looked for a sailboat with a cabin which would give our girls an escape from the sun's heat and berths for all four of us. The San Juan sailboat, locally designed and manufactured, suited the area's sandy beaches and shallow inlets as the centerboard could be raised, and we could cruise coastlines or beach the boat at night. Also, the boat could be parked on a trailer at the club and avoid the more expensive slip fees. We purchased a used, 21-foot San Juan and in so doing had a new master. The strength of the wind or the lack of it controlled how far from the marina we'd sail or where we'd go. The amount of wind determined what, when or if we ate, what we'd wear, who was on board, where we'd sit, and what we drank.

We sailed whenever we had vacations from school and work. One Easter weekend, when Molly was four and Emily, two, we sailed to uninhabited shores where for four days we didn't see any other people. The weather was pleasant, and the girls didn't fight too much. During the days, we found sun-bleached sand dollars dotting the beach. In the evenings, after dinners of kid-food – hot dogs or macaroni and cheese – we skinny-dipped in the river made sparkly by moonlight reflected off the ripples. At night, Tom anchored the boat so that the off-water breezes blew cool, mosquito-less air. Then he'd launch into the adventures of Freddie the Fish, a character of his invention, whose escapades often mirrored experiences the girls had had that day. Freddie the Fish stories were as integral to overnight sailing trips as were anchoring and snuggling into sleeping bags. And after the girls would fall asleep, Tom and I would drink wine and make love on the deck under a canopy of stars.

The distant sky was an ominous black streaked with gray that Easter Monday morning, the fourth day of our vacation. We watched black clouds build as the wind picked up, and the temperature plummeted. To keep warm, Tom sailed in full rain gear while I stayed in the cabin holding the girls to keep them from banging into the sides of the boat or the centerboard wench when Tom tacked. I wished we were in the harbor and not sailing through the storm, but Tom was confident it would pass and kept telling us that we weren't in any danger. It was that confidence that attracted me when we were dating, and was an asset, for the most part, throughout our long marriage and especially during storms at sea when he'd sail and I'd pray while water splashed into the cockpit. Our small boat rocked so much that Easter Monday that all I could see through the portholes was water on one side and sky on the other. In an hour, the worst of the storm was over, and Tom needed a break, so I took the tiller.

The view is always different after a storm, maybe because I'm grateful we've come through it with no damage to ourselves or the boat. The sky that had turned black so quickly was full of light fluffy clouds swirling in the last of the storm's wind. The shade, Carolina blue, is the color of the sky after a storm. The color has a freshness of renewal and a depth that is limitless. It is a color of hope. The white caps disappeared, and the boat leveled. The water's surface, generally glassy after a storm, was streaked with what looked like ribbons of seaweed. As the boat glided past one of the dark, knobby streaks, I saw a fish, a sturgeon, skimming barely under the water looking for food churned up by the choppy waves. Then I realized they were everywhere, as far as I could see, long streaks, some as great as 14 feet; they covered the river. Traveling parallel to the shoreline, they resembled a crew regatta, a sight I had never seen before, or since.

On another weekend trip when the wind picked up, we were with our friends the Sellers whose daughter, Jennifer, was one year younger than Molly and one year older than Emily. As our two boats pulled out of the marina, the girls squealed with delight as they spotted a stowaway, a tiny emerald-green tree frog hugging the mast. As the strength of the wind increased, Preston waved and pointed to a break in the trees and pulled his O'Day ahead of us. We followed. The inlet he led us to was nestled under tall loblolly pine trees that broke the wind. The farther up the inlet we sailed, the gentler the wind became until we found ourselves drifting silently into a world of nature unlike anything on the river. Osprey flew to and from nests perched high in trees. Water moccasins dangled from tree branches that hung above the creek. Primitive gar fish moved through the water with the grace and sound of cinder blocks being tossed from the bank. We could have touched their scaly yellowish-green backs as we drifted past the big fish. Soon the wind calmed and we went back out to the river.

Those and others were the sailing experiences I brought to my boatload of students and Roberta that second summer after Sarah and Kate's first summer. I pointed to the patch of loblolly trees on the far bank as my father had for me, and told the woman sitting next to me, 'That's where we are headed. You adjust the tiller and mainsheet to keep the boat going there. Here, try one at a time. Take the mainsheet and pull it in.' The boat heeled, tipped to the leeward side, the side away from the wind. Uncomfortable tipping the boat, the novice sailor let the main sheet out and the boat rocked back to its level position. 'Now take the tiller and do the same thing. Push it away from you,' I said. She pushed it to windward and the sails fluttered then flapped loudly and the jib sheets snapped against the metal stays of the mast. The new skipper immediately brought the tiller back toward her, and the sails filled with wind, stopping all the flapping. 'Now check your course, I told her. Where is that patch of loblolly trees?'

In the two hours we were out that first evening, each student took a turn at the tiller and the mainsheet. Before the first month ended each woman could operate the outboard motor, find where the wind was coming from, set a course, handle the tiller and mainsheet, and raise and lower the sails. They will never know what they did for my confidence and my ability to trust myself again.

Before the class ended most women learned to sail the wind. When the wind was not steady or very slight, or somewhere else, we'd alter the boat's course to catch the wind. When the wind was too strong, we'd reef as we did the first night out, and we'd lose our ability to point as close into the wind as we might have liked. By sailing the wind we might not have gotten where we intended as quickly as we wanted, but we were moving forward. The wind was out of our control, like a lot of things in life; still, I told them, when we're on the water, we must sail it.

22. Justice must be served

Tom's company offered him a job in Mississippi, so when Kate was three and a half months old we moved bringing our sailboats with us. After living in Mississippi for a while, we realized we were not sailing our San Juan enough to warrant keeping it, as we were too far from water, and we all had busy schedules with school and after-school activities. So we sold it and used the money to visit my family in California. At my Aunt Pat and Uncle Frank's house in Walnut Creek I asked my Uncle Mike, a lawyer, 'If the doctor did nothing and his patient died, did the doctor do anything wrong? I mean, can a wrong be one of omission as well as commission?'

'In the sense of a tort? A legal wrong?'

'Yes.'

'Of course. The doctor's profession is to heal.'

'Cases like these must be filed quickly, right?'

'There is no statute of limitations for wrongful death.'

Wrongful death. The neonatologist was wrong. Sarah's death was wrong. The crime was aptly named, I thought.

At home, I visited with Ray, a lawyer and a friend. 'There are lots of angles to consider,' he told me, 'but one is that of worth. What's a baby worth? A baby dying isn't like a provider dying. A baby is an expense. So you haven't lost monetarily. Now if you had a brain-damaged infant and you could prove negligence, you'd have something because caring for that child would cost money.'

'But the hurt. The grieving over the preventable death of a child. What's that worth?' I asked him.

'It's difficult for juries to measure.' He rested his foot against a drawer of his grandfather's roll top desk, leaned back in his wooden swivel chair, and glanced out the window picking facts from memory and years of legal research. Then he said, 'With all the press that malpractice insurance claims get, and the skyrocketing costs of malpractice insurance, you'd think that doctors get sued all the time, wouldn't you?'

'Sure.'

'Guess again. Most people don't sue their doctors, even if the doctors screwed up. One in 20 hospitalized people is a victim of medical malpractice. That is, one in 20 are injured as a result of medical errors. Of those, maybe one in 65 people will sue. And only 26 will win any damage awards. Doctors, not plaintiffs, win most malpractice cases.'

'Is that why more people don't sue?'

'Not mainly,' he said. He explained that there are a number of other reasons. Doctors and nurses can gloss over the injuries. They might say something like: 'In cases such as yours, this is expected.' What that really means is: 'We made a mistake, but we're not going to admit it to you.' So the patient doesn't get much information or gets distorted information from the only people who know what happened. Most people don't pursue legal action after getting glossed-over explanations from their doctors. Plus, it takes a lot of time and money to prepare a case – about $100 000.

Further he said that childbirth personal injury cases have the worst odds of getting a decision in favor of the plaintiff. And that it takes about ten years from filing a case to settling it. 'They'll try to wear you down by dragging it out,' he said.

'Did you ever have a drink while you were pregnant?'

'Alcohol really makes me sick when I'm pregnant. No.'

'So, you must have sipped alcohol to know it makes you sick when you're pregnant.'

'I don't remember sipping alcohol. Even the smell of it is nauseating when I'm pregnant.'

'Not remembering is all the doctor's lawyers need to accuse you of negligence,' Ray said. 'If you – the person harmed – is found negligent, then the court calls such action "pure contributory negligence" and your damages are reduced. In Mississippi, if you're 50% at fault, you lose 50% of the awards. So, you're on the witness stand, and the doctor's lawyer says: "Mrs Vigour, how can you accuse a doctor of malpractice when you, knowing the health risks to the unborn child, consumed alcohol?"'

'But you're twisting things. The doctor is on trial. I'm not.'

'So you think,' Ray said. 'Everything that the plaintiff does, did, thinks, thought, is on trial. The doctor has lawyers who make it their life's work to beat malpractice claims. The doctor's professional reputation and his livelihood are on the line. Medicine is a powerful and wealthy club, an old boy network.'

'But I told him that Sarah was not premature, and he treated her as if she were premature. Why shouldn't he have to pay? Why shouldn't he be criticized for not listening to me, for misdiagnosing her condition?'

Ray agreed that he should have to pay for misdiagnosing her condition, that justice should be served. But he wanted me to know that I would be up against not just a man but a professional organization complete with attorneys and insurance companies. They will do anything not to lose. Continuing education for them is taking a course in beating malpractice cases.

'The neonatologist was adamant that we not have an autopsy. He even called me at the funeral home to tell me. How would not having an autopsy help him?'

'Evidence. Without it, there is no definitive cause of death. An autopsy also pinpoints the doctor's negligence.'

'I had a dead baby and no one knew why. Do you think he knew he had done something wrong in the way he cared for Sarah?'

'When the neonatologist told you not to have an autopsy performed, he was not motivated by guilt,' Ray said. 'The doctor just didn't want to be caught. Without evidence, there would be less chance of his being caught. He wanted the baby buried along with any evidence that could be used against him. The legal system is in place to stop people like him from making incorrect diagnoses, especially in cases like yours with fatal outcomes. The sad thing is that he'll just keep on hurting people unless he's stopped. A medical license gives a doctor the right to practice medicine; it doesn't say he or she will, or even must, practice good medicine. You could sue for punitive damages on grounds of gross negligence,' Ray said.

The first time I met the neonatologist, we were in his office, and he didn't offer me a seat. So I stood. Molly and Emily stayed behind me, popping their heads out to look at him while clinging to my dress. He kind of barked when he asked me why I was there, saying that he only sees infants and children. I told him that I had a few questions and some things I wanted to discuss with him about the baby I was to deliver. He tapped the eraser end of his pencil on his desk while holding it between his thumb and forefinger. He didn't say anything. He just kept tapping, so I continued talking. Rather than even ask for breastfeeding on demand or ask to be allowed to feed my baby before the milk comes in – so he or she would get antibody rich colostrums – I just told him that I wanted to go home as soon as possible.

'What's the matter? Don't you have any health insurance?' he asked.

I explained that we had good coverage through my husband's company. And that our other two children were healthy at birth, so assuming this baby would be also, I just wanted to go home after he checked the baby. I told him we lived in another town, but I would be delivering the baby in this town and that I wouldn't need his services following the hospital stay.

'But you *do* want me to examine the baby?' he asked. Rising above his remark I just said yes, but my gut reaction was to find another doctor. With only three weeks until the due date, I decided to put his personality aside and trust his expertise. Since Sarah, I trust my gut more.

I impart on him a humanity that I did not see but I must imagine. He had never seen a newborn with group B strep, I imagined. He might have diagnosed her with respiratory distress syndrome. He might have said, 'Sarah was a classic case. I'd seen RDS thousands of times. Only she didn't respond to the treatment as all the others had. She was not the first baby I lost, nor the last, but her diagnosis was one I was sure of. The rapid breathing, the grunting. Classic prematurity.'

'Group B strep. Only two questions out of a hundred on the pediatric board exam and three out of a hundred on the neonatology board exam. The rarity of it takes it off the radar screen. Yet it's underreported.'

'All my mothers get antibiotics now if they come in with ruptured membranes. And all my sick newborns get antibiotics until cultures come back identifying their problem.'

'Would she sue? Sure I wondered. You always do. Her ob didn't think she would, but it didn't change the two-year wait. Jeez. You go into medicine to help. Each diagnosis is based upon ten years of specialized training and more than twenty years' experience. You get 3000 babies with respiratory distress syndrome and one presents with the same symptoms and it's GBS. It was a sad case. The ob told me that she'd had infertility problems. Your whole professional life is geared to improving the quality and length of life. Yet fatal outcomes happen. And when they do, they chip away at you and harden you at the same time. I'm not sure how to explain that. The list of things I can't explain grows.'

Ray called me later. 'The statute of limitations in North Carolina runs out after two years. I'm not sure what your uncle was referring to when he said there is no statute of limitations for wrongful death. Check with him.'

I didn't. Time was past for filing a lawsuit. During the two years I could have filed, grief consumed all my energy. I'd had none left to fight.

If I had tried to serve justice, right a wrong, and thereby, maybe, save other babies, change hospital and doctor policy – would suing have been like the strike at Tom's plant? Labor should have won, but management had more money and power and filet mignon. Yet, the disease is preventable. I might have won.

23. The stone sculpture

In the fall when Kate was two years old, I enrolled full time at the University of Mississippi to finish the last three semesters of a journalism degree. Before Sarah, I was scared that I'd be in competition with students who had not taken a break from their studies and therefore knew far more than I did. But after facing my worst loss, I wasn't afraid of losing or failing anymore. I didn't fail; I did well and went on to get a couple more degrees.

While on the Ole Miss campus that first semester, I noticed an art exhibit as I walked between the journalism building and the student parking lot. The show's paintings, screened prints, and sculptures were bizarre and beckoning. Splashes of reds, oranges, blacks, shapes demanding to be noticed, and designs that swirled or jutted, repelled or moved me or left me staring in amazement. I didn't see the gray stone carving as I first rotated around the room, but once I saw it, every other piece of art revolved around it. The stone sculpture became the hub of a many-spoked wheel of colors and shapes. The piece was small, no bigger than a large overturned cereal bowl, cement colored, drab really with its sparse detail, but the feeling it generated was electric. Chiseled into the stone were the backs of a man, a woman, and three children of various sizes. They were dressed plainly enough to be every man, woman, and child, Anglo Saxon or African, or Asian or Hispanic, or Indian. The heads of the larger figures were touching. Their arms were around each other's shoulders. Days later when judges picked the winners of the art exhibit, the stone sculpture won the award for best in show.

I asked a friend, an art student named Janis, if she knew the sculptor who carved the little family. She did. 'The artist is the wife of a visiting scholar. He is lecturing in the engineering department for a year,' she told me. 'She speaks only Chinese.'

'Would you ask her if she would sell me the sculpture?' Janis said it would be better if she found an interpreter and arranged for me to meet the artist and ask her myself.

Two weeks went by, then a month, and Janis still hadn't been able to set up the meeting. 'I'll pay anything,' I told her. I was obsessed.

My friend arranged a meeting in the artist's studio, and, finally, I was able to meet the artist. She was young, petite, Chinese, with long and very black hair. She didn't speak, but her face was animated with smiles and tiny eyes that laughed.

The stone sculpture was on a table by itself. 'May I touch it?' I asked through the interpreter. The artist smiled hearing my question. The interpreter nodded, yes, I could touch it.

I caressed the stone sculpture, and I embraced the agony of a family surviving the death of a child. I wondered if she had had a child who died. 'Do you have any children?' I asked her through the interpreter.

She shook her head, no.

'Have you ever had any?'

No again. Perhaps her family hugging her before she left China was her model for the piece.

'Your piece was untitled in the art show. Have you titled it yet?'

She shook her head. I didn't tell her, but I knew the name of the piece. It was *Grief*.

'Will she sell it? I will pay anything she wants,' I told the interpreter while envisioning it on my bedside table where it would be the first thing I'd see in the morning and the last thing I'd see at night.

The artist moved quickly around her studio pointing to screened prints of magnificent running horses, mountains, flowers, Chinese landscapes, big pictures hanging high from the hangar-height ceiling. She sorted through yards of oil paintings, pulling out ones to show me. I told her that her work was stunning, that her art would make her famous and wealthy. Hearing my praise, the young artist became like a spinning top whirring around her studio, her black hair whipping behind her as she moved to show me more paintings and sculptures. The reason for our meeting, my request to buy the stone sculpture, continued to go unanswered. Finally, I asked the interpreter, 'She doesn't want to sell it, does she?'

'No. She spent nine months carving it. She will, however, make you a ceramic impression. Would you be interested?'

'Absolutely,' I told the interpreter while seeing in my mind the shapes of the family members in the pearl finish of ceramic glaze.

I visited her studio about once a week over a period of several months. Either she was not there or the ceramic impression was not ready yet. Then one day her paintings and sculptures were gone. A janitor swept scraps of paper, chunks of clay, and dust into piles. 'Where is she?' I asked.

'Who?'

'The artist. The woman who worked in this room?'

'China. She left last week.'

In the language of art, the little sculpture says to hold on tightly to each other when the waves of grief threaten to pull you or someone you love under. It also says when the waves subside, and they do, to support each other's dreams. It says, too, that after you have grieved for someone you loved, you embrace life as you never could before. And we do. With the encouragement of family, I write and teach writing; Tom started his own forestry consulting business; Molly became a lawyer and Emily a pediatrician. And

Kate, the nurturer, the one we all 'mothered,' is quick to reach out to people who are lonely, need tutoring, or are disappointed; she almost recognizes needs before the needy one does. Kate is a chemistry teacher who inspires young people, especially girls, to love the science.

'So you were only going to have three kids, right, Dad?' Kate asked once in the way children ask questions as they piece together where they fit in to the world and what they believe in.

Tom continued reading his book and responded, 'Yeah.'

'Well, that means if Sarah had lived, I wouldn't be here.'

'I guess not.'

Sometime later, when we were alone, Kate asked me the same question. How she figured that Tom and I had decided on a number, I can only marvel. Children discover their parents' thoughts, hopes and demons beyond our imaginings, as we did our parents. 'Ooh, no,' I told her, 'we would have kept trying until we got you. No matter what.' Which got me thinking of life without Kate. Unimaginable. I will always miss Sarah. Maybe I will always see a young girl or woman who is about the age Sarah would be and wonder if Sarah would be as pretty or as smart a dresser or as quick to smile. Maybe whenever I see hair the color of mahogany, I will continue to think of Sarah. But I will always be grateful for Kate. She is an inspiration. She remains kindhearted and optimistic and, like her sisters, has integrity. Even though she's had setbacks that have caused others to give up and give in, like fibromyalgia, which began attacking all her connective tissue at age 11, she has a depth of character, a resilience, a reserve, an appreciation of life and all its possibilities that I've only seen in people older than she who have faced hardships head on, as she has, as we have.

Afterword

In 1990, nine months after her son died of group B strep, Gina Burns of Chapel Hill, North Carolina, started the Group B Strep Association (GBSA) to educate people about the disease, to promote prevention through routine screening, and to promote the eventual development of a vaccine. Parents whose babies died or were injured because of group B strep joined the association; the mailing list swelled to 4000, and after Burns opened a GBSA website, she was receiving 10 000 hits a month. Fueled by anger and outrage, the members banded together to educate and to change legislation. They wrote letters, prepared television and radio announcements, wrote flyers, attended conferences, and published articles in regional and national newspapers and magazines. One group member, a law student, could not find any articles about the legal implications of failing to screen for the disease, so he wrote one saying that failure to screen prenatally for group B strep is medical malpractice. GBSA sought support from prominent researchers and physicians who formed the association's medical advisory board. The grass-roots organization changed the doctors' 'don't look, don't know' policy that had existed for almost 30 years.

In 1994, due to the urgings of GBSA volunteers, legislation was passed in California calling for the state's Department of Health and Human Services to hold a consensus conference to address the issue of testing and/or treatment to prevent group B strep.

In 1996 the Centers for Disease Control (CDC) published guidelines for the prevention of early-onset group B strep disease in newborn infants: to screen mothers and to treat those mothers at risk. The guidelines were the result of six years of effort by the GBSA volunteers, including a letter-writing campaign that produced 5000 letters. The guidelines are not binding; they didn't need to be because GBSA had made the public aware that group B strep is preventable. Pregnant women began asking to be screened. Now screening is routine and deaths due to group B strep have plummeted. The guidelines do not protect all babies: not those who are born before a pregnant woman is tested or those babies whose mothers colonize after the test at 35–37 weeks.

'The rate of early-onset cases', says a CDC publication, 'has decreased from 1.7 cases per 1000 live births (1993) to 0.5 cases per 1000 live births (2000). Since active prevention began in the mid-1990s, the rate of group B strep disease among newborns in the first week of life has declined by 70%. The direct medical costs of neonatal disease before prevention were $294 million annually.'

Mine was one of the 5000 letters sent to the CDC. I wrote about how smart Sarah's sisters are and how much they contribute to their communities whether it be as dorm supervisors or aerobics teachers or math tutors or sailing teachers. Had Sarah lived, I told the CDC, she, too, might have been just as much an addition to her community. One family's loss became a community's loss because of Sarah's potential.

I asked Sharon Hillier, PhD, the director of Reproductive Infectious Disease Research at Magee-Women's Hospital in Pittsburgh, Pennsylvania, why she thought it had taken 30 years to test for such an easily detectable and treatable disease. She said, 'If white, middle-aged men died of group B strep, a vaccine would have been developed in the 1970s. Pre-term deaths and the deaths of babies are undervalued. The money for research isn't there for women's and children's healthcare. Women need to be good healthcare consumers. They need to ask questions.'

Appendix

Sources for information about Group B Strep

ARGENTINA
www.prevencionegb.com.ar (Spanish)

CANADA
La Fondation Canadienne du Strep B (French)
www.strepb.ca

The Canadian Strep B Foundation (English)
www.strepb.ca/home.htm

THE NETHERLANDS
www.ogbs.nl/

UNITED KINGDOM
Group B Strep Support
P.O. Box 203
Haywards Health
West Sussex
RH16 1GF
www.gbss.org.uk/

UNITED STATES OF AMERICA
Group B Strep Association
P.O. Box 16515
Chapel Hill, NC 27516
Email: bstrep@mindspring.com
www.groupbstrep.org

Group B Strep International
East Coast USA Office
61 Carver Road
West Wareham, MA 02576-1227
USA
Tel: 508-273-7247
Fax: 909-620-5557
Email: info@gbs-intl.org
www.groupbstrepinternational.org

Group B Strep International
West Coast USA Office
11 El Dorado Court
Pomona, CA 91766
USA
Tel: 909-620-7214
Fax: 909-620-5557
Email: info@gbs-intl.org
www.groupbstrepinternational.org

OTHER RESOURCES
A Place to Remember
www.aplacetoremember.com

BabyKick Alliance (reduce the risk of stillbirth)
www.babykickalliance.org

Centering Corporation
www.centeringcorp.com

First Candle
www.firstcandle.org

MISS Foundation
www.missfoundation.org

SHARE
Pregnancy and Infant Loss Support, Inc.
National Share Office
St. Joseph Health Center

300 First Capitol Drive
St. Charles, MO 63301-2893
USA
Tel: 800-821-6819 or 693-947-6164
Fax: 636-947-7486
Email: share@nationalshareoffice.com
www.nationalshareoffice.com

FURTHER READING

The Bereaved Parent. Harriet Sarnoff Schiff. Penguin Books, 1978.

Life Touches Life. Lorraine Ash. New Sage Press, Troutdale, OR, USA, 2004.

The Worst Loss. Barbara D Rosof. Owl Books, NY, USA, 1995.

When a Baby Dies. Irving G Leon. Yale University Press, 1990.